THE HEARING-IMPAIRED CHILD IN THE ORDINARY SCHOOL

ALEC WEBSTER and
JOHN ELLWOOD

CROOM HELM
London • Sydney • Wolfeboro, New Hampshire

©1985 Alec Webster and John Ellwood
Croom Helm Ltd, Provident House, Burrell Row,
Beckenham, Kent, BR3 1AT

Croom Helm Australia Pty Ltd, Suite 4, 6th Floor,
64-76 Kippax Street, Surry Hills, NSW 2010, Australia

Reprinted 1986

British Library Cataloguing in Publication Data

Webster, Alec
    The hearing-impaired child in the
    ordinary school.
    1. Deaf—Education—Great Britain
    I. Title II. Ellwood, John
    371.91'2'0941 HV2716

    ISBN 0-7099-3629-X
    ISBN 0-7099-3630-3 Pbk

Croom Helm, 27 South Main Street,
Wolfeboro, New Hampshire 03894-2069

Library of Congress Cataloging in Publication Data

Webster, Alec.
    The hearing-impaired child in the ordinary school.

    Bibliography: p.
    Includes index.
    1. Hearing-impaired children — Education — Great
Britain. 2. Mainstreaming in education — Great Britain.
I. Ellwood, John. II. Title.
HV2716.W43 1985   371.91'2   84-23682
ISBN 0-7099-3629-X
ISBN 0-7099-3630-3 (pbk.)

Printed and bound in Great Britain by
Biddles Ltd, Guildford and King's Lynn

CONTENTS

FIGURES

TABLES

PREFACE

This book has been written primarily for the ordinary class-teacher who has no specialist qualification or experience in teaching the hearing-impaired child. It is intended to provide a comprehensive guide to deafness, and to relate the developmental, social and psychological implications of childhood deafness to situations and experiences likely to be encountered in the ordinary school. The focus of attention is on what the class teacher needs to know technically; the kinds of strategies which enable the hearing-impaired child to learn more effectively in the mainstream; and how the teacher can evaluate the process. This is a source book of practical information about the special needs of hearing-impaired children at all stages of education. It is not a book about integration *per se*, although it encompasses recent developments in philosophy, legislation and research. This work has been made possible by the dedicated efforts of colleagues: specialist teachers, psychologists and speech therapists. We owe a special debt to the Deafness Research Group at Nottingham University, and to those who helped in one way or another with the manuscript: John Bamford, John Crompton, Chris McConnell, Ellen Bown, Jean Gilson and Marianne Wojtan. Our greatest debt is owed to the parents, children and teachers from whom we continued to learn.

Alec Webster
John Ellwood
Kidmore Clinic, Reading

1 INTRODUCTION: THE CHANGING PICTURE

This book has arisen from an in-service training programme developed for ordinary classroom teachers. By 'ordinary' we mean teachers with no specialist qualification or experience in working with hearing-impaired children. The question could be asked 'Why bring this group of children into focus at this point in time?' We will be responding to this question in several ways. At the time of writing there are some significant changes in the wider area of special education in the United Kingdom as well as technological developments which affect the hearing-impaired more specifically.

Many teachers will be familiar with the Warnock Report (DES, 1978); whilst local authorities are currently working through their legal responsibilities to children with 'special needs' as the 1981 Education Act becomes implemented. In terms of legislation the United Kingdom is a number of years behind countries such as the USA, where Public Law 94-142 was passed in 1975 to enable all handicapped children to be educated within 'the least restrictive educational setting'. Consequently, the implications of integration, or 'mainstreaming', of hearing-impaired children in ordinary schools have been much more deeply discussed in the USA than in the UK (Ross, 1982).

The Principle of Integration

We take integration to mean the process by which all children, whatever their abilities and needs, participate together in a community such as the school. The wider debate in special education proceeds along two fronts. First, should the principle of integration be pursued at all? This is a matter for society to decide, and the sociological perspective has been pursued recently by Barton and Tomlinson (1981). These authors are sceptical that the 1981 Education Act, by itself, does anything other than 'nod favourably' in the direction of greater integration of children with special needs into the ordinary school, and will not change underlying attitudes. However, the 1981 Act is a significant milestone, if only because it provides the legislative framework whereby a changing perspective can be openly debated and enacted upon.

For the hearing-impaired the question of integration is more

1

complex than it seems. Many people handicapped by severe deafness identify themselves as a community. An integrated educational programme, where no special methods such as sign language are used, has the aim of preparing children for life in a *hearing* community, not a 'deaf' one. So the policy statements of educationalists (such as the British Association of Teachers of the Deaf) might be totally at variance with those representing the adult hearing-impaired (such as the British Deaf Association). Those who wish to see further discussion on this principle of integration are referred to Booth (1983).

The second question which the wider debate in special education has addressed, concerns *how* integration can be achieved. In this book we have given the issue of principle little space, except to say that the general direction in which special education appears to be leading is towards much greater involvement of the ordinary school in the education of children with difficulties. Where local initiatives are taken to help a child with special needs, then the school requires practical support. Hearing-impaired children are highlighted in this controversial and changing picture partly because of medical advances which have reduced the numbers of children with *severe* sensory handicaps, and partly because improvements in diagnostic techniques and hearing-aid technology have reduced the impact of deafness at *source*.

The trend towards providing for children with less severe hearing-impairments in units attached to ordinary schools (DES, 1967) seems likely to gain further impetus in the present climate. It should be noted that for some years before the 1981 Act many children with substantial hearing-losses have been receiving their education in ordinary schools. This distinguishes them from other groups of special needs children who may have received some form of segregated provision. We shall be arguing that local education authorities need to provide as wide and flexible arrangements as possible in order to respond to the educational needs of individual hearing-impaired children and the expectations of their parents. The 1981 Education Act, at the very least, grants parents the right to ask for their child to be considered for placement in the local school. That may mean, in some instances, considering the diminishing group of more heavily handicapped children for mainstream integration.

It is increasingly likely then, that non-specialist teachers will be aware of children with hearing-impairments in their classes. This raises some fundamental questions. How much information should the teacher have about the nature and implications of deafness?; what practical strategies need to be adopted to help the child make effective use of his learning experience?; and not least, how does the teacher evaluate the learning process?

The Special Needs of the Hearing-impaired Child

What are the educational needs associated with deafness? We know that children affected by relatively mild conductive hearing-losses related to upper respiratory tract infections and congestion, have learning difficulties in school (Quigley, 1978). There are well-documented effects of middle-ear conditions on the child's speech and language development, listening skills, behaviour, reading attainment and general achievement in school (see Dalzell and Owrid, 1976). We have dealt with conductive losses at some length in this book because many children with the condition are not identified and the classteacher is in a good position to recognise the symptoms and be alert to the ensuing problems.

Hearing-impairments caused by some kind of permanent damage to the sensori-neural systems usually have much more serious effects on the child and his caretakers. The most obvious relate to mastering communication and verbally related skills such as reading and writing (see summaries in Conrad, 1979; Quigley and Kretschmer, 1982). Recent findings suggest that the problems are much greater than restricted auditory experience and can lead to wider developmental implications such as social adjustment and emotional immaturity. Deafness is not simply a deprivation of sensory input, but also a disruption of adult-child interactions and relationships (Wood, 1982). Many of these issues we will be dealing with in a practical sense in the separate chapters on classroom methodology.

The Incidence of Hearing Handicaps

It is a surprise to many teachers to know that approximately 1 in 5 children will have a mild hearing-disability at some point in their school careers (Murphy, 1976; Shah, 1981). This figure refers to children affected by conductive or middle-ear problems. Figures for the incidence of hearing-impairments caused by sensori-neural damage are more systematically recorded. In January 1983 local education authorities in England reported that there were 4,040 moderately hearing-impaired children receiving, or awaiting special education. The prevalence rate was 4.88 per 10,000 of the total school population. There were 3,268 children reported as having more severe hearing-losses, a prevalence of about 4 per 10,000 (DES). The decline in the incidence of hearing impairments in children is shown in Table 1.1, which gives figures from 1974 to 1983. Over the decade the trend appears to be a gradual but spasmodic reduction in numbers. This is more marked for severely handicapped children until very recently when numbers of more moderate losses also falls from a peak in 1979.

Table 1.1: Deaf and Partially Hearing Pupils 1974-83 (DES)[c]

| | Deaf | | Partially hearing | |
	a	b	a	b
1974	3,813	4.23	5,202	5.78
1975	3,978	4.39	5,226	5.77
1976	3,968	4.36	4,952	5.44
1977	4,100	4.51	5,509	6.05
1978	4,168	4.63	5,578	6.19
1979	3,905	4.29	5,779	6.35
1980	3,630	4.06	5,310	5.95
1981	3,471	3.98	5,029	5.77
1982	3,387	3.98	4,261	5.01
1983	3,268	3.95	4,040	4.88

Notes:
a. Number of handicapped children receiving education in special schools, designated special classes in ordinary schools, boarded in homes, receiving education under section 56 of The Education Act 1944 (in hospitals, other groups, and at home); and awaiting admission to special schools.
b. Prevalence of above, per 10,000 of total school population.
c. This table is reproduced with the permission of the Controller of Her Majesty's Stationery Office. It is taken from the Department of Education and Science Tabulation of returns on Forms 21M and 7 (Schools) and Table 1 of Consultative Document SH(82)3: 'The Need for Rationalisation of Special School Provision for the Hearing Impaired', June 1982, and statistics from the same sources for 1982 and 1983.

One factor which these statistics do not take into account and which might have a significant impact on numbers of both severely and less severely handicapped children, is the population of children fully integrated into mainstream classes, but perhaps receiving support from a peripatetic teacher. Children whose principal handicap is not hearing-impairment are also excluded.

The Changing Picture

We can look to improvements in medical care to account for the most obvious changes. The immunisation of teenage girls against rubella, therapeutic abortion for pregnant women exposed to rubella, advances in the care of mothers and babies before, during and after birth, all should be reflected in a diminishing population of congenitally hearing-impaired children. There is, of course, no room for complacency. If severe hearing-losses are occurring less often in our children they will be harder to find and our screening and detection procedures need to be as watertight as possible. Great changes have taken place too, through technological developments in the field of audiology. The assessment and diagnosis of hearing-loss depends upon a mixture of objective information and clinical insight. The audiologist and the medical practitioner will work together in this respect. But techniques in audiology have grown vastly. We can now use computer links both for early screening of babies in their cots, and for objective measurements of hearing through electrical impulses recorded in the brain. Similarly, the design and efficiency of hearing-aids and the advent of aids using radio signals rather than sound waves, has brought clearer and more meaningful sound to even the most heavily hearing-handicapped child.

In real terms, fewer severely hearing-impaired children, more sophisticated hearing-aid technology, and a changing economic, social and educational climate, have resulted in several major rethinks. Ten years ago in the education authority within which the authors work it was a commonplace occurrence for severely hearing-impaired children to leave their homes at four years of age in order to join the residential school community for the 'deaf'. The paradox is that despite fewer numbers of severely hearing-impaired children, we are *more*, rather than *less*, likely to meet them within the ordinary school.

Arguments for The Local School

One of the rethinks concerns the 'where?' of education. Should the education of children with handicaps and special needs *necessarily* take place separately from the learning environment of normal school children? The Education Act of 1981 and the underlying research and concepts which went into it, suggests not. Good schools are felt to feed on and give back to the local community, especially at the primary level. Children and families establish friendship groups within their neighbourhood. This is an especially important meeting point for many ethnic minority groups whose children seem to be able to forge lasting understanding and friendship links, where the parents cannot.

There are very special reasons why it is important for a hearing-impaired child not to lose all contact with his peer group. It may well be thought that for a particular child to develop useful speech the best school environment is one where other children have normal speech and where there is rich and pervasive verbal interaction. Parents are sometimes particularly concerned that a child with a handicap is approached with the same expectations teachers have of normal children. Certainly, easy and ongoing contacts between home and school are more difficult if a child has to go away to a residential school, and there may be unavoidable emotional consequences when a child lives away from home and does lose contact with the neighbourhood and his friends. There is too, an important social experience for normal children of befriending a child with more obstacles to negotiate than themselves. Deafness, by its very nature, isolates. We should think carefully, in whatever steps we take, that we do not reinforce that process.

When Integration May Be Difficult

It seems ironical to say that for some children attempts to 'integrate' into ordinary classroom situations may increase the child's sense of isolation. There are many reasons why this should happen. Some lie with the child. There are many children who need to be taught in small groups where individual attention, encouragement and direction can be given. These educational needs are not specific to the hearing-impaired. Such a child may be less 'special' and experience a greater sense of 'integration' being taught alongside other children with similar needs. Nothing diminishes a child's confidence and self-respect more than being a mere onlooker in a group of children far more capable than himself, where the pace and level of work is simply overwhelming.

We are rather more concerned with the ways in which schools and teachers can increase or overcome the problems of isolation which a child's handicap may bring. A very clear illustration of this point comes from one of the author's contact with a visually impaired child. In the ordinary school where she was 'integrated' this visually handicapped child found enormous difficulties in moving about the school, walked into people and doors, fell over steps and wastebins, and on one occasion split her head open on a cupboard door which had been left open and had to be taken to hospital for stitches. Subsequently, the child became 'special' in the sense that all the other children led her about, got out of her way, and either moved objects or shouted warnings to her. In schools where *all* the children have visual handicaps the environment is just as dangerous and full of pitfalls, but the children learn how to cope with it. They avoid walking into cupboard doors, not because there are none, but because they learn how to be independent and negotiate obstacles safely. It is a complex question which of the two school experiences is more 'special' or 'integrated' than the other.

The point we wish to make is that if children with handicaps such as deafness, are going to be taught in ordinary schools, there needs to be much thought and discussion of the practical issues involved. In the example of the visually handicapped child just given, the ordinary school could and did change the way in which the little girl was treated, and helped towards far greater independence. For the hearing-impaired too, the way in which teachers approach their task makes the difference between a meaningful and a meaningless experience for the child. This is, of course, a quite separate issue from the underlying question of whether children should be in special schools or ordinary schools, and that is not an issue we shall be addressing in any depth in this book.

The Need for Flexible Provision

For many hearing-impaired children there will be strong views about the kind of education thought to be appropriate and where this should take place, well before the child reaches school age. Local authorities are often stuck with the arrangements they have, in terms of special schools or units for the hearing-impaired, and the machinery for change moves very slowly. For other hearing-impaired children local education authorities may be rather more predisposed to find flexible solutions to meet special needs. If we are to accept the principles outlined in the 1981 Education Act, which we shall be discussing in Chapter 6, then we should not be trying to fit children to schools, but working out individual arrangements best fitted to each child. Similarly, the question of how well placed a child is educationally needs frequent and ongoing review.

The possibility of a child with a sensory impairment such as deafness, attending a mainstream school is, of course, but one of a range of options, and we do not intend to plead for one kind of provision against another. Many professionals continue to hold the view that severely hearing-impaired children need intensive teaching by specially trained staff using sign language or other methods including 'oral', from an early age. Certainly, some children will have additional learning handicaps quite apart from deafness, which necessitates very carefully prepared teaching and living environments. In some families there are insurmountable obstacles in a handicapped child living at home. So there are many reasons why parents and their advisers may suggest that a child would benefit from a day or residential placement in a special school for the hearing-impaired.

Educationally, the issues revolve around the child's personality, his ability and readiness to learn, his confidence in relating to normally speaking and hearing children, his communication skills and needs, whether he requires the protection and security of small groups and the presence of other hearing-impaired children, whether the child can cope with the demands of a situation where allowances for deafness and anticipation of the difficulties associated with it, are more or less taken for granted.

Questions to be Asked about Integration

Some of these issues are discussed further in the books by Hegarty and Pocklington (1981, 1982). For those children who enjoy some integrated experience one thing is very clear: integration is an umbrella term which means different things to different people and covers a multitude of practices. 'Integration' for one child may mean a visit to a comprehensive school with a specialist teacher for a cookery lesson once a week from base in a residential school for the hearing-impaired. For another child 'integration' may mean that he or she attends a special class full-time which is located in or on the site of an ordinary school. At the other extreme a child might participate *entirely* and without additional help in a normal classroom experience. In between the two extremes are hearing-impaired children who spend some time in units and in normal classes, or who have a specialist teacher for individual help in some subject areas but not in others. Some teachers sit alongside the child in the normal class, others withdraw them.

There are questions to be asked about all varieties of integrated experience. Is it merely locational? Do children share out-of-classroom activities such as eating, play and after-school? How much is the special child participating in and contributing to the life of the school in real terms? There are other relevant issues too, such as how far the main school sees 'integration' as its own problem rather than just the child's. The point which the Warnock Committee's report (see Chapter 6) has made is that ordinary schools already have something like 1 in 6 of their children with special needs of one kind or another. It comes down to a question of attitude and flexibility where one draws such a line: some schools have always been prepared to adapt to the needs of a wider variety of children, others not.

To reiterate, the important issue is that 'integration', whatever that may entail, is not an end in itself. In a good local authority the range of opportunities open to a hearing-impaired child will be varied and flexible, and the drawbacks or points in favour of the various ways of meeting a child's special needs will be discussed openly with the families concerned. But in the end, it is what the child is going to learn which is the important educational objective. Issues relating to evaluation of the child's experience are pursued in greater detail in Chapter 6.

Speech or Sign?

For a severely hearing-impaired child, learning to speak is perhaps the single most important key which can enable him to participate more fully with his peers and family. It is our belief that if a child's hearing-loss is diagnosed early enough, using modern hearing-aids and with good management, then the child can be encouraged to make the best use of whatever hearing he has towards developing speech. We know of many children who have overcome the most appalling hearing-losses to acquire intelligible speech. Some of these children have very dedicated families and teachers who have worked together so that the child can comfortably and meaningfully take his place in a hearing society. The principle we adhere to is that the child is a better learner of language than we are teachers. For this reason we expose him to as much linguistic interaction as possible to ensure that the child's in-built capacity for language is exploited to the full.

We are not so naive as to believe that this can be achieved for every hearing-impaired child. Some children will find speech, even with lip-reading, a most inaccessible code of communication which they could never master. Another of the major rethinks concerns the 'how?' of education. Should children develop sign languages: either by formal teaching in a signing community, or spontaneously themselves in order

that they may converse and interact with their peers? Some authorities believe that the development of normal speech can be supported
by certain signing methods. The 'how?' and 'where?' questions are to
some extent linked in that schools which use sign systems are often
residential. For the ordinary class teacher without any special training,
signing is not an overwhelmingly relevant issue. However, some form of
signing is used with more severely hearing-impaired children in a small
percentage of units in ordinary schools, more often at the nursery or
primary level. Lessons in signing may be offered to ordinary classteachers. It is not beyond the bounds of possibility that signing inter-
preters will be present in ordinary classrooms in the United Kingdom,
although this is not current practice.

Why then have we suggested that signing is not an overwhelmingly
relevant issue for the non-specialist teacher? The position may change
in the future, but the consensus professional view is that if the hearing-
impaired child's needs are so special that he requires an esoteric means
of communication, these needs are probably best met in a special
school where the whole body of teaching and ancillary staff are fluent
in sign language.

Suffice it to say, therefore, that there has been and still is, a great
deal of controversy and emotional argument about the various
approaches used in the education of hearing-impaired children. The debate
has come to be known as the 'Hundred Years' War'. It revolves around
the question of whether sign language can help or hinder a child in his
development of normal speech. What can you do if a child is frustrated
in his need to communicate, when he has little oral speech? Then again,
if a child is taught to sign will he ever see the need to use his voice? The
issues, self-evidently, are very complex, and the research data which
exist are inconclusive (see summaries in Meadow, 1980; Mindel and
Vernon, 1971).

Thankfully, it is enough for most ordinary teachers to be aware of
the issues. Unequivocally, we feel that the ideal for the child must be to
share the normal spoken language which is used by most people as they
go about their daily lives. Anything less is a compromise, but com-
promises are sometimes inevitable. Many hearing-impaired children may
be overwhelmed, even with a specialist teacher close at hand, in the
busy classrooms of a normal school. Some would argue that hearing-
impaired children are happier, make friends more easily and learn better,
when taught in special schools where all the children are hearing-
impaired, where there are dedicated and specially trained staff,
and where there is complete acceptance and awareness of

children's deafness.

Occasionally, a child may suffer more than one handicap: he may have hearing-impairment, visual disability, and be intellectually slow to learn. For this very needy child his parents and teachers may want to try every means of fostering the child's social, educational and particularly, language development. It is unlikely that the special needs of this child could be met in the ordinary school. There is a continuum of special need with many children falling within the two extremes. The 'where?' and 'how?' questions for some children are not easily resolved.

There are schools, however, which offer an environment often described as 'Total Communication'. This is where normal speech, together with lip-reading, a sign system, and a method of spelling out some words by letters on the fingers, are all used as and when appropriate. Such environments are exacting in terms of staff commitment and training, and are usually associated with residential education. Again, it is important that the non-specialist teacher should be aware of these facts and the debate which surrounds them, although they have little to do with the day-to-day events in the ordinary classroom.

The Education Act, 1981

The British government has recently introduced new and complicated legislation about children with special needs of one kind or another, but particularly, educational needs. As a broad rule-of-thumb, the new legislation will apply to those children who have learning difficulties which require additional help to meet their needs which is not normally available within the ordinary school. The definition is open to some interpretation. But children who need to attend a special school because of a physical disability or who are visited frequently by a specialist such as a teacher for the visually impaired, or who need to attend a special class for intensive speech therapy, will be covered by the new Act. Many of the hearing-impaired children in ordinary and special schools will be subject to the new procedures, which bring many changes to the rights of children, their families and their teachers.

Broadly speaking, the Act makes a welcome plea for regarding children as individuals. It is these individual characteristics which education should be concerned with, rather than emphasising the category of handicap with which the child is labelled. We will have more to say about the 1981 Education Act, how provision should be tailored to individual needs and not vice versa, how local school resources are to

play their part in helping to integrate the handicapped, what consti-
tutes good practice regarding 'integration', and not least of all, how
parents and families are to be far more fully involved than they are at
present in deciding what is right and good for their children. All these
things now have the force of law, and there are now statutory obliga-
tions, statutory notices and rights of appeal. New procedures always
seem complex and confusing, if not threatening, but they were designed
to help and protect the child and his parents, first and foremost.

The various advances and changes of the last few years will make
their impact on two important groups of people most of all. First,
'parents as partners' will sound less like a catch-phrase and more like a
responsibility for the future. So, parents should be more closely
involved in what is happening to their child in school. Secondly, the
various rethinks in education, the new legislation, the technological
improvements in hearing-aids, have made it all the more likely that the
ordinary classteacher, without any specialist training, will come into
contact with a hearing-impaired child. That may in fact be an under-
statement. The ordinary classteacher may well be expected in certain
situations to be responsible for the major proportion of a severely
hearing-impaired child's education, to plan appropriate teaching objectives, and to evaluate the overall education experience at the end of the
day.

Help, advice and support for the ordinary teacher vary enormously
from one area to the next. Many teachers will find themselves for the
first time asking: 'How do you talk to a hearing-impaired child?'; 'What
do the facts of her deafness really mean?'; 'Which is the best place to sit
him in my class?'; 'What do I know about radio-aids?'; 'How do I know
whether she can read this or understand that?'. This book is written for
the teacher who wishes to know more about hearing-impairment and
what that means in terms of the practical classroom setting. We have
deliberately avoided contributing further to the emotional debates
about the 'where?' and 'how?' of educating the hearing-impaired. The
issues are mentioned, but we have no particular axe to grind. The fact
is that a number of changes, pressures and reviews, have meant that
'deafness' is an issue which must be faced by many ordinary classteachers for the first time. Whatever the reasons which have brought
this about, the teacher's own needs for information and practical advice
must be met.

Finally, a brief word about terminology. We have assumed that
many readers know little or nothing about hearing-impairment and will
be coming to the subject as beginners. Others may already know a great

deal. Wherever possible, therefore, we have avoided technical jargon where simple language will suffice. We have been concerned to make the complex issues readily accessible to the intelligent lay person. Throughout the book we have used the term 'deafness' to refer to the condition of hearing-disability. It is worth noting that there are very few children who have no measurable hearing at all. The quality, severity, and therefore the impact of deafness, vary greatly from one individual to the next and cannot be predicted. Throughout the book too, we have preferred to describe children *themselves* as being 'hearing-impaired' rather than 'deaf', although the latter is still used, for example, in official documents. Many people feel the latter has emotive connotations and overtones (mostly negative), and betrays a lack of understanding. We have no wish to add to unhelpful controversy. Above all else we have written this book because of our own optimism and confidence in the new developments for hearing-impaired children, their families, teachers and schools.

2 DEAFNESS: SOME BASIC FACTS

The major concern of those involved professionally with the hearing-impaired in schools will be the implications of a child's sensory loss. We must, however, begin at the source. It is often assumed that all hearing-impaired children have the same characteristics and can be considered together as a homogeneous group. We set out, therefore, to explore the complex ways in which deafness can arise, the different kinds and degrees of hearing-loss, and the widely varying implications these may hold for the individual affected.

Teachers will immediately raise questions of a child with a hearing-loss: 'How was it caused?'; 'How serious is it?'; 'Can it be treated?'; 'How was it discovered?'; and 'What does the audiogram mean?' In this chapter we give a brief overview of the basic facts. There are several good textbooks on the aetiology and diagnosis of deafness which offer more technical insights for those who wish, such as Martin (1978) and Ballantyne (1977).

The Normal Ear

It is easier to understand what can go wrong and how we find out that something is wrong, by starting with the normal ear and how it works in health. Figure 2.1 shows the basic structures divided into three sections. It is important to distinguish these sections of the outer, middle and inner ear. Much of what we have to say about the break-down of the normal system concerns the interplay of the three areas involved.

When an object such as a car horn, drum, violin string or a person's voice produces a sound, it does so by causing the air to vibrate in a particular way. Sound is quite simply vibrations in the air. When we shout instructions to our husbands, wives, children or dog, our vocal chords make the airwaves vibrate in a vigorous way and the signal is transmitted through the air. At the other end the signal has to be received. All kinds of receivers, of which the ear is one, have the job of collecting signals. The next and most complex step is to make sense of the information received. We have so far been talking about sound signals in the air. There are many more systems such as radio and TV

Figure 2.1: The Three Sections of the Ear and Types of Hearing-loss

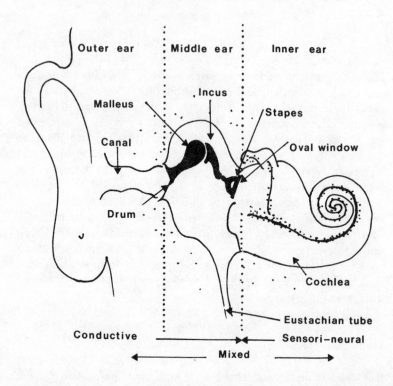

which work on other kinds of signal, but the ear is solely designed to pick up signals transmitted from a vibrating source through the air by means of variations in air pressure.

The shape of the outer ear which we can see and feel on the side of our heads is so designed as to pick up and channel sound vibrations from the air into and along the outer-ear canal. The sound vibrations meet the eardrum at the end of the ear canal which in turn vibrates.

On the other side of the eardrum is the middle-ear cavity, the middle section on the diagram. This is an air-filled space in the bone of the skull. The job of the middle ear is to pass or conduct the incoming sound vibrations across the middle ear until they reach the cochlea at the other side of the cavity. The mechanisms for this are tiny and complex, and consist of three very small bones which are linked one to the other across the air space. The vibrations pass from the eardrum to the malleus, which is fixed to it, then to the incus, and on to the stapes.

The little bone called the stapes is next to a structure called the 'oval window', which is the last stop on the route to the cochlea.

One other feature of the middle section of the ear to draw attention to is the tube which ventilates it, known as the eustachian tube, and which connects the middle-ear cavity to the nose and throat. We can normally feel the effects of the eustachian tube in operation when we swallow. Swallowing opens up the tube to allow air into the middle ear. We need to do this every now and then in order to equalise the air pressure on both sides of the eardrum. If the eardrum is to work like a drum it has to be able to move and vibrate freely. It would not do so if there were differences of pressure on one side from the other.

The third section of the ear, the inner ear, is by far the most complex. The cochlea itself is a tube coiled up like a snail's shell. It is sensitive to the vibrations delivered at the 'oval window', and converts this information into electrical impulses. These nerve impulses pass along the auditory nerve to the brain. It is at this point that the auditory information, the 'message', is made sense of, and a decision may be made to do something about it, to respond. It may be confusing to go into further detail about the complex mechanisms of the cochlea. Certain aspects are worth noting. First, specific parts of the cochlea tube are sensitive to different *pitches* of sound. For example, the cells sensitive to high-pitched frequencies are gathered in the basal turn of the cochlea tube, and the neurones innervating these basal hair cells are found in the outer layers of the eighth nerve bundle. If these are damaged, hearing for some high-frequency pitches may be lost. So too for other specific areas of the cochlea and the sound frequencies to which they are more sensitive.

What Can Go Wrong?

A problem in any one of the three sections of the ear which we have outlined may lead to hearing difficulties. It is by no means uncommon for something abnormal to be happening in more than one structure of the ear, and in some cases all three sections of the ear are working abnormally. Some degree of deafness will result from any difficulty which prevents sound waves from entering the ear canal, from being conducted effectively across the middle ear, from being transmitted by the cochlea in terms of electrical signals, or from being perceived by the auditory nerves and the brain. The extent to which the hearing is affected and the quality of hearing experienced by an individual varies considerably with the structures of the ear which are working ineffectively or damaged. However, the most important distinction which needs to be made is between 'conductive' and 'sensori-neural' hearing losses.

Generally speaking, a conductive hearing-loss is less severe in its effects. Any difficulty which affects the passing or conducting of sound into the ear and across the middle-ear canal may be referred to as a conductive hearing problem. Many kinds of conductive difficulties are amenable to medical or surgical treatment to improve or restore the hearing. The more severe effects on hearing are caused by 'sensori-neural deafness'. Any difficulty which arises in the inner ear, affecting the cochlea, auditory nerve or brain, may be referred to as a sensori-neural hearing problem. The child's hearing is permanently damaged and medical science as yet cannot offer any surgical treatment or repair.

Outer-ear Problems

A few conductive hearing difficulties originate at the very first structure in the three sections of the chain of hearing mechanisms: the 'pinna' or outer ear. Some children are born with malformed ears, no outer ear at all, or no ear canal for the sound to pass along. The latter is unusual, although there was a high incidence amongst 'thalidomide babies'. Without an external ear or canal the problem for hearing sensitivity is that the sound waves are not channelled efficiently into the inner mechanisms of the ear. The inner mechanisms may be perfectly normal and a surgeon may be able to help by creating an outer ear, canal or drum.

Wax or foreign bodies in the outer ear may also cause conductive hearing problems. Wax is, of course, a normal secretion which is usually soft enough to find its own way out of the ear. In some people, however, a hard plug of wax collects in the ear which can swell up with water during swimming or washing. Some children suffer from over-zealous mums who inadvertently compact the ear wax by trying to remove it with special cotton implements bought for the purpose. The dampening effect of compacted wax on one's sensation of hearing may be similar to putting one's fingers tightly in one's ear. Small children have been known to put glass beads, pebbles, marbles, and even dried peas in their ears, much to the concern of their parents and doctors. Where the cause of the problem is mechanical, a blockage, it may be possible to restore normal hearing by removing the obstacle, so long as no further damage is done in the process.

Middle-ear Problems

By far the most common condition associated with conductive hearing loss in children is *Otitis media*. The overall effect of this condition, again, is a mechanical one: the eardrum and ossicles are prevented from vibrating freely in response to sound waves. The sound waves, therefore, are not transmitted efficiently across the middle-ear cavity. In many cases the problem is associated with an infection of the upper respiratory tract. A child may typically suffer nose, sinus and chest infection or have a 'catarrhal cold' and the adenoids may become enlarged. There are important consequences of this because the adenoids lie at the base of the eustachian tube which is short and more horizontal in a child. If the eustachian tube becomes infected and is prevented from working properly, a whole chain of events may follow.

In the first stages of the condition air already in the middle-ear cavity is gradually absorbed by surrounding tissue. The air pressure within the cavity becomes negative relative to the air outside, which has the effect of sucking the eardrum tightly inwards. Stretched and taut, the eardrum is no longer elastic enough to vibrate freely in response to sound waves. If the eustachian tube blockage persists and the middle-ear cavity is unventilated, a watery fluid is produced in the middle-ear space. Fluid in the middle ear affects the free movement of the tiny ossicles as they attempt to pass on sound vibrations. Hearing problems caused by thin fluid can be intermittent and come and go within a few days. This makes it disconcerting for parents and teachers to decide whether a child really does have a hearing difficulty, when the evidence for it seems to fluctuate so much. Very often children are more affected in winter when there are more infections about, than in summer months. Catlin (1978) suggests that about a third of children who develop fluid in the middle ear have a history of allergies. In some children, when secretory *Otitis media* has gone untreated for a long period, the fluid becomes mucoid in consistency. The eardrum and ossicular vibrations are severely dampened by the thick exudate. This condition, often likened to running in a swimming bath, as opposed to through the air, is commonly called 'glue ear'. It is difficult to say how many children suffer from significant conductive hearing problems in the early years of school. Some authorities estimate as many as 20 per cent, but how many of these children are diagnosed and treated is the pertinent question.

Treatment of Otitis Media

Fortunately, *Otitis media* is usually amenable to medical treatment. The GP can often diagnose a middle-ear infection by observing the condition of the eardrum. A course of antibiotics may be prescribed to clear up the infection, or a decongestant to dry up the sinuses and eustachian tubes.

There is also surgical treatment for middle-ear problems if other methods have failed. The surgeon may remove tonsils and/or adenoids if they are blocking the eustachian tube or causing repeated infections. A surgeon may wish to draw out any fluid from the middle-ear cavity by making a tiny incision in the eardrum. If it is felt that adequate ventilation might still not occur after removing fluid and there is a chance that the condition may begin over again, a 'grommet' may be inserted into the eardrum. This is a tiny 'teflon' tube which allows air to pass into the middle ear through the hole in its centre. This treatment has been likened to opening a window in a damp bathroom in order to dry it out. Until recently grommets did not remain in the eardrum for very long and usually came out of their own accord while the hole in the drum healed over. A new T-shaped grommet now in use is designed to stay permanently in the drum until removed by the surgeon. In the past children particularly prone to fluid in the middle ear may have needed it drawn off and grommets inserted several times during childhood. While the latter may no longer be necessary, it is still important that parents and teachers do not assume that once a child has been treated for a middle-ear problem, then he or she is necessarily cured. Conductive hearing difficulties of this kind may well recur, and some signals to look out for are repeated infections, colds, catarrh, mouth-breathing, snoring, and of course, signs that the child cannot hear so well (see Appendix I).

Chronic Otitis Media

This is a more serious kind of middle-ear condition. The problem here is the risk of damage to the eardrum or ossicular chain caused by longer-term infections. In many children *Otitis media* occurs acutely. Inflammation arises suddenly and causes much discomfort. It is at this point that a caring parent will take the child to the doctor: the moment that earache is complained of. The child's discomfort, given antibiotics, may disappear quickly. Some parents may be inclined not to finish the course of antibiotics in the mistaken belief that the infection has cleared. Certainly, many parents never return to their GPs to check. An infection which remains in a subacute state may not be painful, but may have insidious effects. A residual infection over a long period may lead to complications such as adhesion, scarring or disease of tissues, which the surgeon may have to remove to prevent further damage. Surgeons are now able to replace parts of the chain or the ossicles if they are diseased, and can reconstruct the conducting mechanisms of the middle ear. Needless to say, ear infections in the early stages should always be treated very carefully in order to avoid subsequent problems of a much more serious nature.

Inner-ear Problems

Conditions affecting the third section of the ear, the inner ear, usually have serious implications for hearing. It is also true, unfortunately, that there is little or nothing that can be done to repair damage of the inner ear. There are many *known* causes of sensori-neural hearing-losses. But for a very large group of hearing-impaired individuals with sensori-neural deafness, the cause remains a mystery.

Table 2.1: Structures of the Ear Involved in the Two Kinds of Hearing Difficulty

Type of hearing loss	Part of ear affected
Conductive	outer ear
	middle ear
Sensori-neural	cochlea
	auditory nerve
	auditory tracts in the brain

Maternal Rubella

An expectant mother who gets rubella (German measles) between the sixth and twelfth week of her pregnancy, may have a damaged baby. This is the time in a pregnancy when the embryo's delicate organs are forming, including the cochlea. A baby affected by the rubella virus before birth may have heart defects, visual-disabilities and brain damage, such is the seriousness of the disease during pregnancy. In certain cases it is thought that the embryo can still be attacked by the virus even if the mother is immune to the disease. Nevertheless, the programme of immunisation for young girls against rubella has reduced the number of babies affected. Many doctors offer abortions to mothers who are known to have had rubella at a critical time during pregnancy. These are some of the reasons why the numbers of severely hearing-impaired children are falling. A few years ago a rubella epidemic meant a certain increase in hearing-handicapped children.

Other Viral Infections

Many other viral infections contracted at important stages of the pregnancy for the growing embryo can cause damage to the inner ear. It is also true that a baby can be infected immediately before or after birth if the mother has chicken pox, measles, even influenza, and a serious hearing-loss may be the consequence.

Anoxia

A difficult labour or a long, complicated birth may mean that the baby is short of oxygen. Lack of oxygen can result in damage to the nerve cells in the auditory pathway causing a hearing-loss. Many maternity hospitals take great care to monitor the baby during birth if the labour is not straightforward and if the baby is 'distressed'. Improved maternal care during delivery is another important reason for falling numbers of severely hearing-impaired children, and there are certainly far fewer babies who suffer handicaps through anoxia than there used to be.

Prematurity

An infant born before having spent the allotted 40 weeks in the womb, is described as premature. Sometimes this term is used of any baby which weighs less than 2.5 kg (5½lb) at birth. There are many risks for premature babies including damage to the nerve cells of the ear. Premature infants are more likely to be injured during birth or to contract infections. They are less robust and therefore more vulnerable than full-term babies.

Jaundice

Jaundice is a blood condition affecting the new-born baby, sometimes because of a mismatch between the blood groups of the mother and child. Severe jaundice can cause damage to the nerve cells in the auditory pathway. Fortunately, it is another problem which is better understood and better controlled in modern hospitals, and nowadays far fewer children suffer from deafness as a result of jaundice.

Meningitis

Meningitis is probably the commonest post-natal cause of deafness in young children. It is an acute inflammation of the covering of the brain which can lead to mental handicap and spasticity, as well as hearing-impairment.

Other Childhood Illnesses

Many of the commonly occurring illnesses of childhood can very occasionally be suffered so severely as to lead to inner-ear damage. Mumps, measles, scarlet fever and whooping cough have all been reported as causing hearing-impairment in children.

Genetic Origin

Many children inherit deafness, and this may even be the case where there is no deafness in earlier generations. That may seem contradictory, but it is possible for individuals to carry the necessary chromosome within their genetic makeup which might produce a hearing-impaired child if the other parent was also a carrier. Such a couple would have a one-in-four chance of having a hearing-impaired child with every pregnancy. This process is known as a 'recessive' genetic tendency. The only hope of reducing the numbers of children with hearing-loss caused in this way is by genetic counselling. There are, of course, many children who inherit deafness directly from one or both parents. It is also perfectly possible for a parent with deafness to have a normally hearing offspring.

Cause Unknown

In any group of children with severe deafness there is always a large proportion for whom the cause is unknown. In many children the cause may actually be recessive genetic, but it is often difficult to prove unless further hearing-impaired children are born to the same couple. In other cases mothers do not always remember a viral infection in the early stages of pregnancy. Symptoms, such as a rash, may have been very slight. Often, anoxia at birth may be suspected as the cause, but there is no real way of knowing. It is, of course, natural for parents to want to know why their child cannot hear. However, it may be extremely difficult to be certain of the cause, especially when events are being seen in retrospect. Often, all that can be given to parents is a probable reason for hearing-loss.

How is a Hearing-loss Identified?

It is extremely important that a child with a hearing-loss is discovered as quickly as possible so that something can be done to help. Sadly, there will always be a few children with severe hearing-losses which go undetected for several years. The early years, when normal children are rapidly acquiring language, are crucial. Severe hearing-losses undiagnosed until 3 or 4 years of age, may have serious consequences for the child's later development. Unfortunately, there will be many children with middle-ear or conductive hearing-losses of a milder nature whose hearing difficulties are never recognised. To the unsuspecting teacher, a child may appear 'lazy', 'disruptive', when in fact he cannot *listen* very easily.

There are many reasons for suspecting a hearing problem, and it is well to know what these are, particularly for children in school. Hopefully, all children with severe sensori-neural losses will have been picked up long before school age, although there are some hearing problems such as high-frequency losses which may not be detected until later. We may well know in advance that a particular family is at risk of having sensori-neural hearing problems. A parent, close relative or other siblings may be known to doctors and other professionals already. Similarly, factors in the family history, or in the pregnancy, or delivery of a baby, may be known which predispose a child to having a hearing-loss. A premature or small-for-dates child, for example, would be carefully monitored for hearing-loss from an early time.

In most areas the community health services organise screening and testing procedures to try to pick out infants who may have hearing difficulties as early as possible. Health Visitors usually endeavour to screen every baby either at home or in the Child Health Clinic, using simple but carefully prepared techniques and materials to see whether the baby responds to sounds. Of course, there are many reasons why a child should fail or pass this screening test, apart from hearing-loss, but if the Health Visitor is concerned about a child's hearing, referral can be made to the child health doctor (Community Medical Officer) whose special concern is audiology, or via the GP to a hospital ENT/audiology department.

Health Visitors watch out for problems of hearing or speech in children up to school age. At age 5 years another hearing screen is usually given in school by an audiology technician or school nurse. Again, if concern is expressed about a child's hearing in school at any time, the school nurse can follow this up and refer on to the specialist child health doctor, if necessary. The next step may be for the child to be seen at hospital for treatment and advice. Alternatively, the family doctor can refer a child to the audiology department at the local hospital at any time if there are worries about a child's hearing. It has to be said that there are bound to be difficulties in co-ordinating all the various services at large in the community, in schools and in hospitals. The level and quality of service offered can vary enormously from one area to the next.

Whatever steps are taken to investigate possible hearing-loss in a child, there should be as little delay as possible. There is one point that cannot be emphasised enough: mothers often *know* there is something amiss with their child's hearing. A mother may sense that her baby of a few months old does not seem to react to sudden loud sounds or to hear her voice. The baby may show no signs of startle at a door slamming or sudden clatter of pans on the kitchen floor. A parent's worries should always be taken seriously and as often as not are found to be justified. A parent should *never* be fobbed off with unfounded reassurances such as, 'he'll grow out of it' or 'he's just slow to talk', by anyone.

For the older child the onset of a hearing-loss, such as a middle-ear problem, may be signalled through falling concentration, inattention and tiredness in school. The teacher may have noticed a tendency to 'mess about' in class rather than listen. A child may frequently seem to be day-dreaming, forget to bring equipment or misunderstand instructions through having misheard. Instructions may have to be repeated several times. A child may not turn immediately when called by name and seems to be much more 'with it' when nearer to the teacher. A child with problems in listening to sounds is also going to have difficulties with early reading methods which depend on building up sounds to make words.

At home the parents may have noticed that a child wants to sit nearer the TV or have the volume up louder than usual. The child may have started to mouth-breathe or snore heavily, and have persistent catarrh and colds. Earache itself is obviously a clear sign that something may be amiss and may need treatment (see Appendix I). Wherever concern is expressed about hearing by a teacher or parent who is in close contact with a child, thorough investigation should be promptly carried out. This will often involve some kind of audiometric test. Different techniques have been devised to suit children of different ages and capabilities. Each ear is usually checked separately because it is possible for one ear to be affected and not the other. All audiometric tests try to give us information about two separate aspects of hearing.

Frequency

It is important to know whether a child can hear the normal range of sounds, i.e. high as well as low pitch. The pitch of a sound is referred to in terms of *frequency* which is the speed of vibration of sound waves measured in Hertz (Hz). Sound waves vibrating very rapidly produce high tone sounds. Slow-vibrating sound waves give rise to low sounds. Speech is produced partly by our vocal chords causing the air to vibrate. It contains a complex mixture of high and low-frequency sounds. Some of the sounds in speech are not made by the vocal chords but by the tongue and lips, such as 's', 't', 'p'. We have already noted that it is possible to have defective hearing for high sounds and normal hearing for low sounds. A child with a high-frequency hearing-loss would have some difficulty in hearing the beginnings and endings of words which are mainly consonants, such as 't', 's', 'f'. On the other hand, the middle bits of many words, usually vowels such as 'a', 'e', 'i', 'o', 'u', have mostly low-frequency components. It is essential to know, therefore, whether a child can hear across the range of sound frequencies, and to test for these separately.

Intensity

The intensity or loudness of a sound is measured in decibels (dB). The loudness of some everyday sounds is given in decibels below.

rustle of a leaf	10 dB	
very quiet speech	40 dB	comfortable listening
normal conversation	60 dB	
vacuum cleaner	70 dB	
busy traffic	80 dB	
shouting	90 dB	causes discomfort
heavy drill	110 dB	
rock band	120 dB	painful
jet engine	140 dB	

It is important to understand that the intervals in the decibel scale are not equal. Because the scale is logarithmic the actual difference between 120 and 140 dB is many times greater than the actual difference between 40 and 60 dB. When a child is described as having a 50 dB hearing-*loss*, this means that sound has to be made louder by 50 dB in order for the child to detect it, compared with a person of normal hearing. A decibel hearing-loss therefore describes the *discrepancy* from normal in the child's hearing. The same child with a 50 dB loss would be unable to hear the rustle of a leaf or very quiet speech, but would just barely detect normal conversation. In testing hearing we will need to know the level of loss at every separate frequency because there may well be important differences.

Hearing Tests

Testing the hearing, particularly of a baby or young child, is not always an easy task. A great deal of skill and experience is required, especially if testing is carried out at a hospital or clinic, where a child may feel anxious from the very start. Testing depends very largely on the child wanting to co-operate and being capable of responding to a signal. We have to be very sure, with tests of all kinds, that it is absolutely clear what the test is revealing. A nervous child, a child who does not understand, or an unco-operative child, may fail a hearing test for reasons other than hearing-loss itself. Traditional tests are often subjective. The audiologist gives the child some form of sound signal in one ear and has to interpret the response which the child makes to the sound stimulus. The most recent developments in audiology have been towards more objective measures of hearing. There have been several attempts to find ways of testing children's responses to sound which cut out human interpretation and error and which can be used as early as possible. Audiology is a growing science and we will be looking at some of the remarkable techniques being developed later in the chapter. For the majority of children, traditional testing will be the norm for some time to come.

Distraction Tests

A distraction technique (Ewing and Ewing, 1944) is often used to test the hearing of babies from about 7 months to 18 months of age. The basic principle is that babies who are able to sit up, with good back and head control, will turn to locate a sound made out of the field of vision. This is the type of test which Health Visitors are trained to use for young babies at 8 or 9 months old. The baby is usually sat on the mother's knee, supported at the waist and in a slightly forward position. The baby's attention is attracted to the front by one of the examiners, perhaps using a toy or ball. The second examiner presents a sound stimulus behind the child's line of vision. High and low-frequency sounds are presented separately at the quietest level consistent with normal hearing. If the baby does not turn then the sounds are made gradually louder until a definite response is observed. A baby who did not begin to turn to high and low sounds until they were presented at a 50 dB level may be suspected of having a 50 dB hearing-loss. The test would usually be done several times, using different sound stimuli, and on each side.

To an observer this test may appear crude and unscientific. Certainly, there are many hazards in carrying it out properly. Conditions have to be quiet, the child must not be too absorbed in what is going on in front of him, the examiner must be careful not to move into the child's line of sight when making the sounds. However, when carried out by skilled and experienced people, distraction testing can give very accurate and reliable results with most children.

Co-operative Tests

Co-operative testing is normally considered appropriate for children from 18 ·months to 2½ years of age. This is not a popular technique because one is relying on the child's co-operation at an extremely *unco*-operative age! The principle here is that most children with normal hearing can follow instructions given by voice at around the 35- 40 dB level. A child may be asked, in a voice of carefully controlled intensity, to 'put the brick on the chair', or 'give the dolly to mummy'. If a child begins to respond appropriately only when a louder voice is used, this may suggest a hearing-loss. It may also suggest that the child does not understand instructions easily, or is unused to doing things which are asked, or is simply inhibited. It is not possible, using co-operative testing, to tell whether the child has hearing difficulties in high, as opposed to low, frequencies, and other testing would have to be done to find this out.

Visual Reinforcement Audiometry

The basic principle of visual reinforcement audiometry is that a child is trained to look in a certain direction wherever he hears a sound stimulus by rewarding him with the sight of an animated toy, illuminated puppet or attractive picture. The technique is useful for children aged from about 6 months to 3 years and may overcome some of the limitations of distraction and co-operative testing. The child is usually seated at a small table and occupied with a toy. A sound stimulus is presented through loudspeakers placed to the left or right of the child. A looking or turning response is rewarded by the brief presentation of a puppet, toy or flashing light, usually close to the sound source. Here too, the child must be co-operative, alert and interested, but the technique provides fairly precise information, for example, about the child's sensitivity to sounds across several frequencies.

Performance Tests

By the age of 2½ years a child is usually capable of completing a performance test. Often the child is involved in a game, such as putting a brick in a box, or a peg in a board. The child is trained to respond to a stimulus (such as 'go') by dropping the brick in the box or fitting in a peg. The test proceeds with the child continuing to respond in the game, but to other signals, such as the high-frequency 's' sound. As in distraction testing the sound is made louder until the child begins to indicate that he has detected it.

Pure-tone Audiometry

A child of 3 or 3½ years should be capable of completing a pure-tone audiogram, and it is this test which is favoured from then on. An audiometer is used, which is an instrument capable of producing sounds at specific intensities and specific frequencies across the range of normal hearing. Sounds are delivered to the child's ears via headphones, and the child is trained or instructed to listen and wait for a sound before making a response. The results of the test are displayed on a chart called an audiogram.

An example of an audiogram showing a severe high-frequency loss is given in Figure 2.2. Along the horizontal axis are plotted the sound frequencies, from low to high, which are sampled during the test. The vertical axis plots the threshold of hearing, the point at which the child begins to respond, at increasing levels of intensity or loudness of the signal. The further down the intensity scale from O dB the child's threshold appears, the greater the hearing-loss. The sound signal has had to be increased by the amount shown in order for the child to detect it. Remember, when interpreting the scale showing hearing threshold, that it is logarithmic.

In the example shown, convention is followed and an 'X' is used to indicate results for the left ear, an 'O' to denote results for the right ear. In clinical practice, responses showing up to 15 dB hearing-loss across the frequency range are taken to be within the limits of normal variability. This audiogram shows a child with a normal response at 250 Hz for the left ear. The right ear has a 20 dB loss at 250 Hz and 500 Hz, which is just outside normal limits. The hearing-loss increases in both ears, the higher the frequencies sampled. The loudness levels of the everyday sounds given earlier can be used to interpret the intensity at which high-frequency sounds would need to be presented to this child in order to be detected.

Figure 2.2: Audiogram Showing a Severe High-frequency Hearing-loss

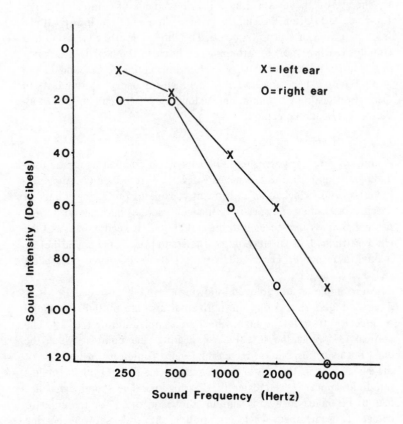

Bone Conduction

This type of test can reveal whether a hearing problem lies in the middle ear, or is sensori-neural in origin. When a pure tone is presented to the child through headphones, the signal travels down the ear canal where it vibrates the eardrum and ossicular chain. The sound waves are converted into electrical impulses at the cochlea and eventually perceived by the brain. The whole system has to be in working order for the pure tone test to succeed.

Instead of pure tones through headphones, sounds can be presented to the child through a small vibrator which is placed on the mastoid bone behind the ear. The signals produced in this way vibrate the skull. This stimulates the inner ear directly through the bone. The mechanisms of the middle ear are effectively 'by-passed'. A normally hearing person should hear the signals conducted through the air and through the bone at about the same levels of intensity.

Figure 2.3: Audiogram Showing a Middle-ear Hearing-loss

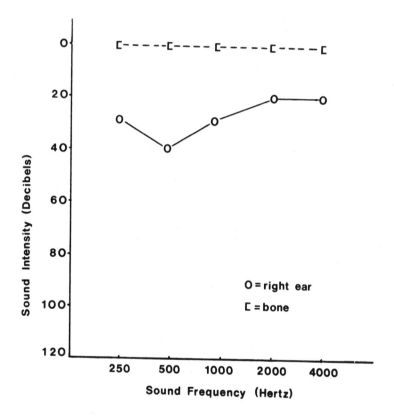

Note: The [symbol indicates that the non-test ear is masked by noise.

In Figure 2.3 the audiogram shows the results of pure-tone audiometry and bone conduction for a child's right ear. The bone transmitted signals (marked by [ ) are within normal limits across the frequency range. However, the pure tone results through headphones indicate up to a 40 dB loss. Since the pathway through the bone to the inner ear is normal, the loss must lie in the mechanisms of the middle ear or outer ear before the sound enters the cochlea. The loss is therefore conductive in nature.

If a child's audiogram showed a loss both for air *and* bone conducted signals then the results of the bone conduction test and pure-tone audiometry would look similar and the loss would therefore be sensori-neural in nature (Figure 2.4).

Figure 2.4: Audiogram Showing a Moderate Sensori-neural Loss

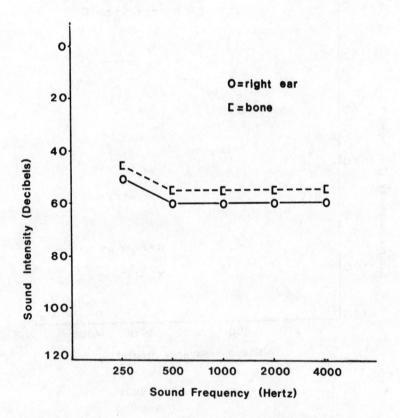

Note: The [symbol indicates that the non-test ear is masked by noise.

It is possible that a child has a mixed hearing-loss involving both the middle ear and the inner ear. In such a case the bone conduction levels would be depressed with an additional loss of sensitivity for air-conducted signals. It is important to realise that children with sensorineural hearing-loss are as susceptible as anyone else to transient middle-ear disorders causing conductive loss. For such a child the effect may be temporarily very serious, reducing what little hearing the child has.

Speech Audiometry

Although an audiogram gives precise information about a child's ability to hear pure tones, it gives only a crude indication of the child's ability to hear spoken language. We have already noted that speech sounds are very complex and cannot be broken down easily into component pure frequencies. Therefore, in order to understand what a child can hear of spoken language it is useful to carry out speech audiometry. When a child comes to be fitted with a hearing-aid to help him use and understand speech, it may be important to have speech audiometric information.

In speech tests the child listens to a voice presented freefield, through loudspeakers or headphones, to lists of phonetically balanced words. More recently, children have been asked to listen to specially constructed sentences which contain representative proportions of the different speech sounds and familiar vocabulary (Bench and Bamford, 1979). The child is asked to repeat what he hears, and a judgement is made about how clearly the child can discriminate between different sounds in speech at different intensity levels. We can also measure to what extent a child can follow normal conversation and how this changes with the loudness of the signals.

'Objective' Tests

All of the techniques of assessment we have outlined require the active involvement of the baby or child. The child has to *respond* in some clear way so that the examiner knows that a sound has been heard. There are many ways in which children can give misleading information about their ability to hear. The most worrying aspect of subjective testing is that some children will pass a hearing test by responding to clues *other than* the sound signal. A few of these children will be hearing-impaired. It would be extremely useful to have alternative ways of assessment which did not depend for success on such human factors as co-operation and subjective interpretation.

The Auditory Cradle

The auditory cradle has been developed to test the hearing of new-born babies in maternity hospitals. It uses a computer to present sounds, then measures and records the baby's responses in the form of changes in breathing and body movements. The computer also has to work out whether the baby's responses during the test are real indications of hearing-loss, compared with the response patterns of a normal infant. The process is automatic. The cradle is still at the stage of being tried out in practice, and is not yet in general use.

Impedance Audiometry

Although not strictly a test of hearing, this technique gives very useful information about the functioning of the middle ear. It measures the amount of sound reflected by the eardrum when a sound wave reaches it. It will be recalled that in some children hearing-loss arises because of negative air pressure and fluid in the middle-ear cavity. The eardrum is unable to vibrate freely as it should in response to the incoming sound signals.

Impedance audiometry uses a very simple technique. A small plastic probe is placed in the child's ear canal for a few seconds. A tube in the probe feeds sound into the ear. A second tube has a microphone which picks up the sound being reflected from the eardrum. A third tube allows the examiner to control the air pressure on the outside of the eardrum. In a normal ear the sound travels down the ear canal, through the eardrum and across the middle-ear cavity. Very little sound is reflected back from the eardrum because normally it is flexible and therefore conducts sound very efficiently.

If a child has a middle-ear problem, such as secretory *Otitis media*, the eardrum becomes stiff, with the result that less sound is conducted across the middle ear, and more sound is reflected back by the drum. This is picked up by the probe and recorded on a chart. The test is objective because the child has nothing more to do than sit quietly and still. Impedance testing enables the examiner to tell whether or not a conductive hearing-loss is present, and gives valuable information as to the likely pathology.

Electric Response Audiometry

It is known that very small electrical changes occur in the auditory nerve and the auditory pathways in the brain when a sound signal is presented to a normal ear. Over the last few years tests have been devised using computers which can measure these minute electrical changes in or near the brain. Electric response audiometry can be used to confirm a suspected severe hearing-impairment with children who are unco-operative or handicapped, and therefore unable to participate in conventional testing.

The scope of these specialised test techniques is limited by expense and availability. Only a few centres are able to offer it in this country. The process may involve the child having a general anaesthetic so that an electrode can be passed through the eardrum to the covering of the cochlea. More often the test is conducted using non-invasive electrode placement when the child is in a natural or sedated sleep. The information which the test gives at present is not very specific. It may indicate severity of hearing-loss but be unrevealing about the frequency pattern involved. Electric response audiometry, nevertheless, is an important supportive means of identifying hearing-impairment.

Many people believe impaired hearing is simply the loss of hearing sensitivity, where sound is not loud enough. It should be apparent that the way in which deafness occurs, how it is diagnosed and what it means to an individual, is far from simple. Hopefully, the incidence of severe hearing-impairments will continue to fall. Ten years ago over a third of the hearing-losses diagnosed were caused by mothers having German measles during the early months of their pregnancies. There is now a programme of immunisation for teenage girls against rubella, and this measure, together with therapeutic abortion and many other medical advances will reduce the numbers of children with severe hearing-losses. We are hopeful too of the new techniques and refinements in the science of audiology for the early detection of hearing-losses. It is true, of course, that if deafness is occuring less often in children it will be much harder to find, and our 'search-strategies' need to be highly efficient.

Hearing-aids

We conclude this chapter with a discussion of the most significant and in some cases, *only* 'treatment' available for a child with servere sensori-neural hearing-impairment: hearing-aids. Since hearing-aids and their use is one of the most crucial aspects for the child we have also dealt with the subject in subsequent chapters, highlighting the most relevant factors at different age levels. Hearing-aids lessen the impact of deafness *at source*. The later a sensori-neural loss is identified, diagnosed and hearing-aids fitted, the more serious the effects on the child's development. The whole thrust of early intervention is towards providing more meaningful auditory experience, by exploiting the child's residual hearing to the full. Hearing-aids do not, however, *restore* a child's hearing to normal. Hearing-aids simply make sounds louder. For the child with profoundly damaged hearing mechanisms, even very powerful amplification may not present the child with much useful auditory information. Nevertheless, there are very few children who derive no benefit at all, and some who benefit greatly, from hearing-aids.

Types of Hearing-aids

In simple terms a hearing-aid picks up sound, amplifies it, and then delivers the louder signals into the ear canal. The basic components of conventional hearing-aids are a microphone, amplifier and receiver (or speaker). Conventional aids fall into two categories: those worn on the body and those worn behind the ear. Both kinds are prescribed free of charge to hearing-impaired children in the United Kingdom. There are many models of hearing-aid available within these two basic designs, each with different qualities and characteristics. Whether a particular aid is selected depends upon the age of the child, the nature of the hearing-loss, the degree of amplification required, and the effectiveness of the aid for the individual user.

Both body-worn and post-aural aids have adjustable settings which make a significant difference to what the child perceives and so the classteacher must understand the controls and be aware of the correct settings for the child. All aids have an on and off switch so that batteries are not wasted when the aid is not in use. The increase in amplification (or gain) is controlled by a numbered or marked wheel and a recommended gain setting will have been made for the particular child. Some aids have tone controls which alter the quality of the output and which will usually also be set. Other settings may limit the output of the aid at certain frequencies and should not be interfered with. In many instances these settings are only adjustable by a jeweller's screwdriver.

Most conventional aids have a control switch marked M, T, or M/T. For normal everyday use the control should be set to the M position, whereby the microphone picks up sound signals in the environment for amplification. If the control is moved to the T setting the aid no longer picks up environmental sound. The T setting indicates a loop coil facility. The T facility by-passes the microphone of the hearing-aid and picks up signals from a magnetic field. A loop system is basically a wire installed around a room and then connected to a sound source, such as

Figure 2.5: A Post-aural Hearing-aid

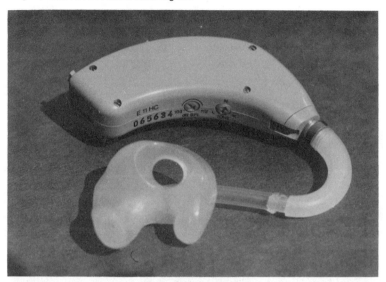

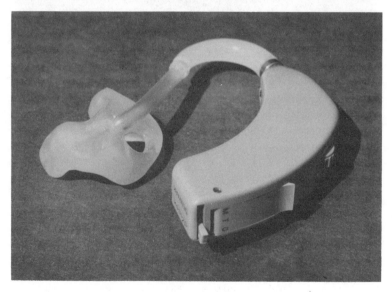

A post-aural hearing-aid with sound tube and earmould. The microphone aperture is visible near the hook of the aid, as are the output and tone adjusters. The M, T and Off switch is located just below the battery drawer, and the volume wheel is placed above this.

Figure 2.6: A Body-worn Hearing-aid

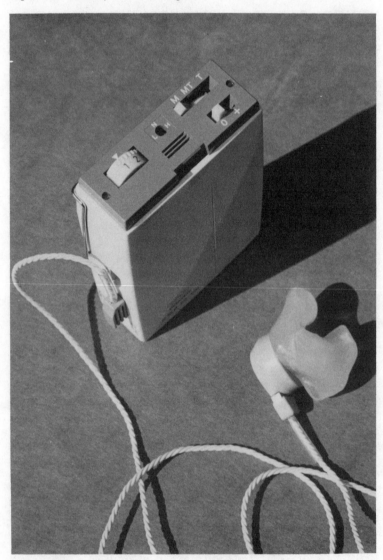

A body-worn hearing-aid with cord connection to the receiver, which is fixed to the earmould. The weak spots on the cord are protected by plastic sheathing at the plug-in points. On the top of the aid the On/Off switch, output limiters, volume wheel, and M, M/T, T modalities can be seen, together with the microphone aperture. The retaining clip is visible on one side, with the battery drawer on the other side.

a television set, which drives the loop. A classroom can be fitted with a loop, which is then driven by a teacher's microphone and amplifier. When the teacher speaks an electric current will pass through the wire loop around the classroom, setting up a magnetic field which varies according to the speech signal. The T facility in the child's hearing-aid picks up the magnetic signals, converts them into electrical signals, which are then amplified and converted back into sound by the aid. Body aids and some ear-level aids have an M/T switch which enables the use of a loop system together with the environmental microphone of the aid.

Body-worn Aids

In the body aid (see Figure 2.6), the case which houses batteries, microphone and amplifier is attached to the child's chest. The receiver is separated from the amplifying system by a long cord and delivers sounds into the ear canal through the earmould. Body aids are sturdier than other types of aids and their controls are easier to manipulate. Because of their size, batteries may last much longer and are easier to change. Body aids are capable of giving powerful, good quality sound amplification across a wide frequency range and are easier to repair. The most important advantage of the body aid is that feedback is less of a problem. Feedback occurs when amplified sound leaks out around the earmould if it is not a good seal, and is then picked up by the microphone of the aid again. The result is a disturbing high-pitched whistle. Because of the greater distance between the microphone (located on the body) and the receiver (located at the ear), the feedback cycle is less likely to occur.

Body aids have several disadvantages. Since they are worn on the torso, the speech signal is not detected at the normal ear position. The body itself will reflect and absorb some sounds, and the microphone of the aid may well be covered with clothing. The rubbing of the microphone against clothes also produces unwanted sound distractions. Body aids are difficult to conceal for cosmetic purposes. The bulk and position of the aid, together with the cords, may get in the way of an active infant. Most parents find they have to secure the body aid in a harness and cover the microphone aperture with a thin film of cellophane to keep it clean.

Post-aural Aids

Post-aural aids (see Figures 2.5 and 3.1) are small and inconspicuous and sit behind the pinna. Since the aids are worn near the normal location for perceiving sounds some of the normal ear's capacity for detecting direction can be replicated. The case of the post-aural aid houses all the components, including battery, microphone, amplifier and receiver, but excepting the earmould. Post-aural aids incorporate highly efficient micro-chip circuitry and provide the same range of amplification as body aids. However, there may be a narrower frequency response and a poorer sound quality than is possible with the larger microphone and receiver of the body aid.

Since the microphone and the receiver are closer together in the post-aural aid feedback problems are much more likely to arise. The controls can be difficult to manipulate. Batteries are expensive and have a shorter life. Wind noise can be a factor with certain aids in the playground on a blustery day. Post-aural aids are more easily lost, dropped, crushed or submerged, and are more difficult to repair. Some children have problems in retaining the aids behind the ear because of the shape or size of the pinna, and parents have to make recourse to sticky tape. Notwithstanding some of these drawbacks, post-aural aids are usually the recommended choice except for very young infants.

A very recent modification of the post-aural aid, which we shall only mention briefly here since few children are currently prescribed them, is the in-the-ear aid. The entire aid, including microphone, amplifier, receiver and battery, is contained within the body of the earmould and, inserted into the ear. The in-the-ear aid is expensive but inconspicuous and neat, with the principal advantage that it normalises the placement of the microphone in the ear and allows the pinna to play its normal physiological role in sound reception. They are not recommended for younger children because of feedback problems and the recurring need to restructure the aid in new moulds as the child's ears grow.

Binaural Amplification

For the vast majority of hearing-impaired children, providing hearing-aids for both ears will improve the ability to comprehend speech and locate a sound source. This is especially true of noisy situations which demand that the child focuses his attention for long periods. Some parents resist two hearing-aids for their child as though he might be considered doubly-handicapped. However, there are only a few exceptional cases where binaural hearing-aids are inappropriate. Children with very marked discrepancies in hearing sensitivity or speech discrimination between their two ears, may be prescribed just one aid. The benefits of binaural amplification are a main reason why post-aural aids are fitted more often than body aids. It is physically much less convenient to achieve binaural amplification with body-worn aids than with ear-level aids.

Earmoulds

The earmould is a vital part of a child's hearing-aid system which channels the amplified sound down the ear canal towards the eardrum. With a body aid the receiver is held into place close to the ear by the mould, and with a post-aural aid the tubing from the receiver is fed into the ear canal. If the earmould is not a good fit the amplified sound can leak out around it, be picked up by the microphone of the aid again, and a high-pitched feedback whistle is produced. In order to achieve a good seal earmoulds are made from individual impressions of the child's ears, and a left mould will be quite different from the right. The material used for taking impressions is usually a soft silicone rubber which is syringed into the ear and left to harden. The second stage involves manufacturing the finished mould from the cast. In a few cases a one-step process is used whereby the impression itself can be used as the final mould. Various materials are used for making earmoulds; in children the trend is towards softer and more flexible moulds. Children need to have earmoulds replaced three or four times a year as their outer ears grow and the seal becomes imperfect.

Some children find the impression-taking process unpleasant, whilst the final mould has to be skilfully made in order to create a good fit. Moulds are occasionally lost, blocked or chewed and are often a source of great irritation, particularly when feedback problems arise. Replacing a new mould on the child's aid is fairly simple. With the body aid the receiver clips into the mould; with the ear-level aid the mould is just placed in the ear, the aid is rested on the pinna, and the plastic tube connected to the mould is cut at about 5 mm (¼ in) past the end of the hook of the aid. The tube is then pushed on to the hook of the aid.

Fitting an Aid in the Ear

Some parents inadvertently try to put the left mould in the child's right ear and vice versa, whilst one individual we know wore the aid itself in his ear, leaving the mould hanging loose. Eventually, even very young children can manage to fit their own aids and to replace the moulds if they become loose. However, teachers should be aware of how an aid is properly fitted, particularly with post-aurals.

If the teacher needs to replace a post-aural aid for a child the first step is to hold the earmould firmly on its outer edge. The mould should be inspected to make sure it is clean and the sound tube free from wax. The mould is then inserted into the ear canal and with a backward twisting movement the mould is then pushed fully into the outer ear. The hearing-aid is then slid over the pinna to sit neatly behind it, ensuring that the sound tube is not twisted in the process. Check the aid is set at the right output level and switched on properly and that there is no feedback whistle.

Taking Care of Aids

Post-aural aids are less robust than body-worn aids, and it is on the occasions when they are taken off that they are most vulnerable to damage. When not in use the aid should be kept in the strong hinged box provided for its safekeeping. It is important that children begin to take responsibility for caring for hearing-aids from an early time, for example, when the child is changing for PE or swimming. Aids should be switched off when they are not being used to preserve the battery life, and if they are to be stored for any length of time the batteries should be removed. Aids left in pockets can be lost, stolen, crushed, put through the washing machine, and in one instance we know, eaten by a dog attracted to the feedback whistle. The most important step that can be taken to care for body-worn aids is to ensure that they are securely harnessed to the child and child-proofed with a cling-film cover.

Testing a Conventional Aid

It is important, particularly with younger children, that the teacher is able to check a hearing-aid to make sure it is working properly. The teacher may suspect, from the child's behaviour or lack of usual response, that the aid is malfunctioning. All children should be encouraged to complain if the aid is not working. However, there are some day-to-day checks which can be made by the ordinary classteacher. A cupped hand over the child's ear should induce faint whistling feedback in an ear-level aid, if it is working. If the aid is taken off and the volume turned to full, there should be a strong feedback whistle. It is a good idea to listen, through the receiver, to the quality of sound the aid produces. This is a little more difficult to do hygienically with post-aural aids, but a plastic stethoscope can be bought to listen to the output of the aid.

Visual inspection will often reveal dirty or loose parts of the system. The mould should be clean and the sound tube free from wax. The tube should not be cracked, crimped or contain condensation. With a body-worn aid the cord should be checked, particularly at the weak points where the cord connects to the aid or receiver. The microphone aperture should be clean and not blocked with food or other spillage. Perhaps the most obvious of checks should be made on the battery. The classteacher should hold a supply of new batteries and know how to replace them, with the terminals facing the correct way. The aid will, of course, only work if it is set to the appropriate controls and switched on.

The centres which supply hearing-aids and some educational services for hearing-impaired children, have hearing-aid test boxes. This specialised equipment tests whether aids are working to their design specifications, by assessing the frequency responses at various input levels and volume control settings. Where there is any doubt about the proper functioning of a hearing-aid, a thorough objective assessment can be made by specialists.

We have summarised in Table 2.2 the fault-finding procedures which the non-specialist can follow. Faults in a child's hearing-aid should be rectified as soon as possible, and both specialist teacher and parents alerted. The teacher of the hearing-impaired may be prepared to leave spare parts, such as a cord or receiver, or a spare aid, with the classteacher.

Some Problems with Conventional Aids

Children and their adult caretakers have to learn to use hearing-aids effectively. Hearing-aids are selected, fitted and adjusted within the sympathetic acoustic conditions of a clinic or hospital. However, situations in which the hearing-aids are actually used may be most unsympathetic acoustically. It is crucial that the classteacher understands the advantages and drawbacks which different listening environments present to the child using conventional hearing-aids. These points are discussed more specifically in the age-related chapters, but it is well to be aware from the outset, that hearing-aids require management strategies.

There are two major factors involved. First, the child's ability to hear with aids depends on distance from the sound source. Secondly, listening skill will depend on the level of competing background noise in the environment. Hearing-aids simply make sounds louder; they do not select from the sounds available in the environment, the most relevant or meaningful sounds for the listener. So, if a speaker is positioned outside the range of peak efficiency for the aid, which is approximately 2 m (6 ft), it becomes increasingly less likely that the voice will be picked up by the microphone of the aid, as the communication

Table 2.2: Fault-finding Procedures for Post-aural and Body-worn Hearing-aids

Fault	Cause	Cure
No sound	Not switched on	Check on/off switch
	Aid set to T	Turn to M
	Dead battery	Replace
	Battery inserted wrongly	Place + to +
	Earmould blocked with condensation or wax	Wash in warm water and dry
	Post-aural: plastic tubing crimped or twisted	Turn mould over
	Body-worn: cord broken or frayed	Replace cord
On/off intermittent signal	Switch contacts poor	Turn on/off several times
	Poor battery contacts	Realign contacts
	Post-aural: tube twisted	Untwist or replace
	Body-worn: poor cord connections to aid or receiver	Manipulate cord/replace
Feedback (whistling noise)	Poor earmould seal	Re-insert
	Poor-fitting earmould	Inform parent/specialist teacher
	Excessive amplification	Reduce volume/check setting
	Body-worn: poor seal between receiver and mould	Replace receiver
Poor sound quality	Weak battery	Replace
	Body-worn: dirty microphone aperture	Clean with soft brush
	Internal fault, e.g. volume wheel	Inform parent/specialist teacher

distance increases. The microphone of the child's aid does, of course, pick up all other sounds in the environment. In a busy classroom situation, if the teacher is trying to say something over a wide communication distance from the child's aids, it is likely that there will be a nearer or louder sound source which the aids will pick up. The noisier the listening environment, the more difficult it will be for the child to listen selectively to the sounds he wishes to hear.

The implications of these factors for classroom practice are important, and teachers should be aware of optimum acoustic conditions, where to position the child to avoid noise interference, and what strategies to adopt to enable listening and communication. In general, high-ceilinged rooms with hard surfaces contribute noise interference because of reverberation. Speech perception is usually better using conventional aids in listening conditions with soft furnishings, carpets and sound-absorbent materials such as cork wall tiles. The teacher must be careful to avoid sitting the child near to sources of noise, such as a well-used play, store or sink area. In each of the age-related chapters to follow we have outlined appropriate teacher strategies for managing communication. In fact, these are mostly designed to normalise what the teacher does, since a common assumption is made that the teacher may need to over-articulate, or worse still, shout at the child. The latter changes normal rhythms of speech and may overload the hearing-aid, leading to a distortion of the output to the listener.

Radio Hearing-aids

The use of radio transmission in hearing-aid systems has effectively overcome many of the problems associated with the communication distance in conventional systems. A radio system comprises a microphone/transmitter unit worn by the teacher and a receiver/hearing-aid worn by the child. We shall be describing several of the various systems currently available. However, the basic process involves, at one end of the system, a microphone suspended or attached to within 15cm (6 in) of the speaker's mouth. The speaker's unit also houses a transmitter with an aerial, which converts the sound input into a radio signal and then broadcasts it on a permitted radio-frequency range. The child's unit houses a receiver (not a hearing-aid transducer, which is also termed a receiver) tuned to the same radio frequency and which detects the signal. At the other end of the system the output from the receiver is amplified by the child's hearing-aids and fed into the child's ears. The speaker's voice is effectively transmitted to the child's aids without interruption to the signal, across distances of many metres if necessary.

Radio Aid and Hearing-aid Combined

In one variation of the basic system the child wears a single unit which is both a radio receiver and a conventional hearing-aid. The child's unit is bulky and resembles a body-worn aid with some of the problems associated with the latter in terms of its conspicuous size. The system can be used as a normal body-worn hearing-aid when the radio facility is switched off; for example, if the child is involved in a group-play activity and direct input from the teacher's transmitter is not required. On the other hand, the child's microphone can be switched off so that radio transmitted signals only are received. This might be appropriate in situations such as school assembly, where background noise is high and the child benefits from a clear and direct signal from the teacher's transmitter. Finally, the system can be used as a conventional hearing-aid and as a radio receiver at the same time. The child receives information from transmitted signals as well as from the environmental microphone on the aid itself which enables the child to hear sounds in his vicinity, including his own voice. There is considerable flexibility of function. The teacher can turn the transmitter on when it is useful to give a clear message directly; and the child retains the use of the conventional hearing-aid when the radio facility is switched off. In fact radio aids must be used selectively and carefully. Not all that the teacher says is relevant to the child wearing the aid, and it is not exclusively the teacher who needs to be heard clearly.

Radio Aid with the Child's Own Hearing-aid

In a second type of radio system a transmitter and receiver are used in conjunction with the child's personal hearing-aids. Again, the radio microphone/transmitter is worn by the teacher. The teacher's voice is transmitted via radio waves, and a radio receiver worn by the child picks up the signals. The receiver is connected to the child's personal aids by a lead to an input socket. The aid must have a direct input facility, usually a plug connection or a shoe which slides over the bottom of the hearing-aid. Not all hearing-aids have this direct-input facility, however. Signals fed into the aid from the receiver are amplified in the conventional way and delivered to the child's ear. The hearing-aid's own microphone also remains sensitive to sound while this system is in use so the child continues to receive environmental sounds including his own voice. The radio receiver can also be disconnected entirely to leave the child's aids, post-aural or body-worn, functioning normally.

Radio Aid with the Loop

Aids without direct input can use this type of system through the loop facility (T or M/T setting). A loop of wire is taken from the radio aid receiver and worn by the child; around the neck in the case of post-aural aids, or around the aid itself in the case of body-worn aids. The radio microphone/transmitter unit works in the normal way in picking up the teacher's voice and transmitting a radio signal. The child's receiver picks up the signal and converts it into a magnetic field via the loop worn by the child. This signal is then converted into an electrical signal by the T coil of the child's personal aid and amplified in the usual way. Where the child's personal aids have an M/T setting the child will be able to hear his own voice and sounds in the vicinity, together with the radio input. However, loop systems used in this way do have some disadvantages. The performance of hearing-aids on the T setting is often inferior to the aid's performance in the normal M mode: the frequency range amplified may be reduced and there may be variations in output. Should an aid not have an M/T setting then the system is much less flexible and the child will be unable to hear the sounds of his own voice in the vicinity, unless the receiver has an environmental microphone.

Fixed Radio Systems

Radio aids can be used not only to drive a small loop worn around the child's neck, but also to drive a wire loop fitted around a room. This would enable a number of children wearing hearing-aids on T mode, to benefit from transmitted signals. In one fixed system infra-red light waves are used to transmit the sound signals. Infra-red emitting diodes are placed high in the four corners of the classroom and the signal is detected by a special receiver worn by the child and utilising the direct input or T coil facility in the child's aids.

Advantages and Disadvantages of Radio Aids

Radio aids have made an invaluable contribution to the successful participation of hearing-impaired children in mainstream classes. By overcoming the problems associated with communication distance in conventional hearing-aid systems, children dependent on aids can receive clear speech signals even in noisy listening conditions. For very young children there is no need to sacrifice freedom of movement and exploration to achieve good amplification of speech signals. The degree of flexibility of some of the available systems is very useful. In some systems it is possible for more than one child to be linked to a common radio frequency in order to receive transmitted signals, whilst other children can be given a personal frequency.

However, the radio systems are comparatively expensive and are not as yet available on the National Health. Some local education authorities are investing in radio-aid provision and maintaining aids bought by charities and parents. Radio aids require careful management and some specialist oversight. Routines need to be established for their care, for efficient use of battery life (8 to 12 hours before recharging), and for exploiting their full potential in the normal classroom. This last point we have taken up in greater detail in the age-related chapters.

Testing a Radio Aid

The specialist teacher of the hearing-impaired should be available to advise on the testing of particular radio systems, but there are some day-to-day checks which the ordinary teacher can make. Obviously, if a radio system is used in conjunction with the child's personal aids, checks should first be made on the child's hearing-aids, using the guidelines already described. It is important to ensure that the correct settings are made and the aids switched on properly. The child should be encouraged to report if the system is not working. The teacher can place the radio transmitter by a sound source in another room, and then listen through the child's aids to the reception quality. The radio-aid units can be visually examined for broken wires, loose connections, or dirt in the microphone apertures. It is, of course, essential that the batteries are routinely charged, and some radio aids are equipped with a warning light which indicates a low battery voltage. Some basic fault-finding procedures which the non-specialist can follow are given in Table 2.3

Table 2.3: Fault-finding Procedures for Radio Hearing-aid Systems

Fault	Cause	Cure
Transmitter	Low battery voltage	Recharge/replace
	Microphone connection	Plug in
	Loose aerial	Manipulate/repair
	Not switched on	Check switch
Receiver	Low battery voltage	Recharge/replace
	Aerial loose/broken	Send for repair
	Loop wire broken	Replace loop
	Different frequency channel	Check frequency code of transmitter and match with receiver
	Volume set incorrectly	Adjust
	Loop/microphone leads plugged in wrongly	Check plugs/sockets
Hearing-aid	Low battery voltage	Replace
	Wrong mode setting	M for direct input T or M/T for loop
	Direct audio-input lead broken	Replace
	Shoe connection wrong way around	Turn around
	Volume not set loud enough	Adjust
	Loop too far from hearing-aid	Adjust

We have provided a basic introduction to the physical facts of hearing-impairment, its aetiology, identification, diagnosis and treatment, including hearing-aids, in the hope that teachers will find this a useful reference resource. However, the physical facts are only the very beginning. The real nature of a hearing-handicap for the child, his family and teachers, is what the remainder of this book is about.

3 FIRST STEPS : PRE-SCHOOL AND NURSERY

In this chapter we consider the very wide implications of a hearing-loss for the young infant and his family. The child's potential for development in terms of social, language and educational achievement, is highly dependent on his early experiences. We shall be examining the nature and quality of the hearing-impaired child's early interactions with others, both at home and in the nursery, well before the child actually begins to talk.

Of all the things we learn, language is probably one of the most important if we are to live a normal life. Language plays an integral part in our thinking and our conceptual growth. Communication fosters social relationships and emotional adjustment. For the child with a severe hearing-loss, learning to speak will be the most critical achievement, and this inevitably tends to be the focus of our efforts in helping such a child. We shall be making a case, as others have done (Chazan, Laing, Bailey and Jones, 1980), for early intervention once a handicap is discovered. We hope to highlight aspects of early management which help children make the most of their residual hearing and encourage language development. The ordinary nursery school can play a key role in supplementing the stimulation provided at home. Hearing-impairment has been described as a 'hidden' handicap in the sense that its consequences are covert. There are several recent summaries of research which show, however, that severe deafness can disrupt almost every aspect of healthy socio-psychological development (Meadow, 1980; Quigley and Kretschmer, 1982; Fundudis, Kolvin and Garside, 1979). In deciding how best to respond to the early educational needs of a hearing-impaired child, there can be no complacency.

Some Early Obstacles

There are several accounts of some of the very real obstacles which parents have to negotiate with a young hearing-impaired child, from those who have first hand experience. In Gregory's (1976) interviews with mothers of hearing-impaired infants, the greatest problems were associated with communication: not being able to explain to a child why he must hurry or wait, what he is permitted to do and why certain rules are followed. Mothers soften the blow of having to go home from a friend's house, to give a toy back, or to finish a game later, through explanation.

We are concerned in this book with a range of hearing-handicaps, and not all of the children we refer to have severe communication problems with their parents. However, we know that even moderate conductive hearing-losses slow down the child's language development (Quigley, 1978) and general readiness for school (Bax, Hart and Jenkins, 1983). So common childhood occurrences like temper tantrums, getting a child off to sleep, toilet training, mealtime behaviour, instilling road sense and awareness of other hazards, all take on additional overtones since they may be more difficult to establish.

We are beginning to discover more, through research, of the disruption which deafness brings to mother-child interaction *before* the child begins to talk. We know that the games which mothers play with their babies such as 'peek-a-boo', or 'this little piggy went to market', have a function. They are the first shared dialogues in which the child takes part. Where a child has auditory impairment, the first 'conversations' between mothers and babies about a shared experience, exchanges involving turn-taking when first the mother and then the baby responds, and anticipation games, are all interfered with and may be missing altogether (Gregory and Mogford, 1981). We are beginning to realise then, that the implications of deafness for a young child are far greater than imperfect hearing of sounds.

Once deafness has been diagnosed in a child the parents will look to the 'experts' for advice. It is difficult to co-ordinate advice given to parents, especially when there are so many agencies involved. In an article written by the parent of a hearing-impaired child, Tumin (1978) suggests that the three most frequent sources of complaint made by parents are: the giving of inadequate information, unrealistic advice, and ignoring what parents themselves have to say.

One area of controversy concerns language. How can we best help a child learn to speak? Parents are sometimes told by early advisers that they will need to *work* on language, to teach every word. Other counsellors suggest behaving as *normally* as possible, to provide the same opportunities and environment as one would for a hearing child. Much of what we have to say in this chapter is an elaboration of the pitfalls involved when those who come into contact with young, hearing-impaired children either over-modify their approach, or make no adjustments at all.

The Teacher of the Hearing-impaired

It usually falls to the peripatetic teacher who has specialist training and experience in work with the hearing-impaired, to guide the family through the first steps after diagnosis. The child with a severe hearing-loss will need audiological assessments, ENT examinations, possibly the fitting of earmoulds and hearing-aids, and the visiting teacher will offer support, guidance and information. The teacher will normally make frequent and regular visits to the child's home from the point of diagnosis until school entry. It is part of the peripatetic teacher's role to co-ordinate the involvement of outside agencies such as medical, audiological, psychological, and to ensure that the most effective sources of help are available without overwhelming the family. Without doubt the most important help that can be given to a hearing-impaired child and his family is the hearing-aid. At all levels in school, non-specialist teachers, together with parents, can look to the teacher of the hearing-impaired for expert advice about hearing-aid management. Very few children have no residual hearing at all, so even the most profoundly impaired child can be helped to utilise what he has. The sooner that amplification is given, the sooner the effects of deafness are reduced *at source*.

Parents often make very close links with their visiting specialist teachers because of the major readjustments which families have to make. The specialist teacher will be dealing with fundamental questions such as 'Will my child learn to talk normally?'; 'How will he relate to other children?'; 'What will happen about schooling?' It is well for those teachers involved at the ordinary nursery or first school stage to know, that unlike most hearing children and families, there has already been heavy involvement with professionals and perhaps, in some families with a hearing-impaired child, the expectation that this will continue.

Why the Ordinary Nursery?

It is widely accepted that by the age of 3 years or so, children with a range of hearing-losses, from moderate to profound, can benefit from *some* contact with a group of normally hearing children. For more severely handicapped children this is likely to be a smaller part of the child's experience, with other time being spent in a special class with a very high adult-child ratio. In the United Kingdom, unless family circumstances are such that the child cannot live at home, it is increasingly less likely that a child will attend a nursery in a special school for the hearing-handicapped, to the exclusion of all else. The changing outlook described in Chapter 1 accounts for some of the underlying reasons for this, and for the rising expectations of parents. The ordinary nursery or playgroup offers children social contact with peers and the opportunity for linguistic interaction enmeshed with the play experience (see Figure 3.1). The hearing-impaired child is exposed to normal speech of children his own age and size, talking at his level, about the things he is interested in. The value of a well-designed and purposeful nursery experience for *all* children has been argued by many writers (Webb, 1974). For the hearing-impaired child the argument is based more centrally on language development.

Figure 3.1: Hearing-impaired Child in an Ordinary Nursery

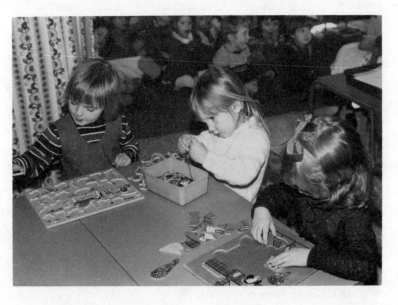

This little girl, happily playing alongside other children in a nursery, is wearing a post-aural aid, which is cosmetically less intrusive.

Since deafness does not affect the child's *biological* capacity for learning language, if he is to use this capacity to the full he needs more exposure to an ordinary speech environment and wide opportunities for play with peers already using language at his interest level. It is in the sense of widening the linguistic interaction available to the child, that a good nursery should supplement, and not supplant, the child's experience at home.

A note of caution is appropriate here: nursery provision varies widely in its organisation, staffing and general aims. A report by Tizard (1975) showed that in some centres staff spent most of their time supervising children or putting out play equipment, and least time talking to the children, suggesting activities or helping children to do things. In nursery schools which had carefully examined how best to stimulate learning, productive play and language, staff inevitably spent more time interacting with children for 'cognitive' purposes. It is the responsibility of those professionally involved with a 'special needs' child, particularly the teacher, to monitor how well an educational experience is meeting the child's specific needs. We shall be discussing patterns of interaction in some detail in this chapter, whilst in the final chapter methods of evaluating the child's interaction with peers and adults are considered. Wood (1982) addresses some of these issues for the more profoundly hearing-handicapped child in an article which highlights that it is not so much the *kind* of educational placement which matters, as what goes on between the child, his peers and his adult caretakers, when he is there.

First Contacts with the Ordinary School

In just the same way as a hearing child needs careful preparation and introduction to his first day at school, so too the first contacts with a group are very important for the hearing-impaired child. For the handicapped child there may be extra difficulties in leaving the security of home. Some hearing-impaired children may be able to attend a local nursery or school, in which case there may be siblings or familiar neighbourhood children who already attend, and the mother will be able to pick the child up herself and have easy contact with staff. For more severely handicapped children it may be recommended that a child attend a specialist facility attached to a normal school, and this is unlikely to be near to home and will involve travelling. Initial contacts and ongoing home-school links need careful thought when this situation arises.

For some hearing-impaired children discussion and explanation of the coming event of the first day at nursery or school will be difficult. Perhaps the most satisfactory preparation is for the parent to visit the group with the child in the term before entry, one afternoon a week for half a term. This can also be reciprocated by teaching staff. In the authority in which the authors work, the nusery teachers in the special units attached to ordinary schools also work as teacher-counsellors and visit the families in their homes. The ordinary teacher in a nursery or infant group where there is a hearing-impaired child could also make this very useful bridge by visiting the family at home.

There are other useful ways in which children can be prepared for nursery or school. Some of these are discussed by Bishop and Gregory (1983). A child might have been encouraged to keep a scrapbook recording important events in the pre-school years. Photographs of the teacher or class, bits and pieces relating to the pre-entry visits, all can be included in a scrapbook which focuses the child's anticipation and gives the future event some real form.

We have already mentioned that the greatest problems and worries expressed by parents relate to communication with their child. When initial contacts between school and home have been well organised, the parents will have discussed with the teacher any individual ways that have developed. The parents have lived closely with their child's growing language and there may be special ways by which the child indicates his needs, such as wanting to go to the toilet, feeling thirsty, tired or hurt.

Attitudes to Deafness

Perhaps the most important first step that the ordinary teacher has to take in coming into contact with a hearing-impaired child is to clarify basic attitudes to the handicap, a process the parents will have already gone through. The child will have some useful hearing, and the focus should be on helping the child to make sense of what he does hear, rather than what he cannot. Once this point is accepted teachers may be inclined to feel more comfortable with a hearing-impaired child. Some teachers say that they feel odd talking to a child who doesn't hear! Of course, many nursery teachers will already have experience of children who are late in developing speech, and the principle of enriching the language input to the child is fundamental to the view that the child is a better learner of language than we are teachers, when the right experience is provided.

Attitudes to Discipline

Hearing-impaired children are very different from one another, if only because of the wide variations in hearing-loss, let alone their unique personalities and experiences as growing children. The 'all deaf children' trap has been used to describe the pitfalls in expecting all hearing-impaired children to behave in the same way, have the same likes or dislikes, abilities and disabilities. Deafness is certainly not responsible for everything the child does. In the book by Cleave, Jowett and Bate (1982), which documents *ordinary* children entering school, aggressive, irritable and defiant behaviour appears, as well as more positive developments. Very little of the hearing-impaired child's behaviour should be thought of as deviant. If demanding behaviour arises and is exacerbated by communication difficulties, the teacher will still want to establish similar boundaries as for any other child. The process may take longer, require more examples and repetition to be given, and the child may need more definite 'black and white' signals. Deafness should not be a reason to allow a child to 'take charge' of the home or nursery group. Like all children, the hearing-impaired child will look for adult approval, encouragement and acceptance. These can only be achieved when limits to behaviour are set by the adult. Where there are communication difficulties with the child, there is a problem of spelling out clearly where the boundaries are. Adult feelings of sympathy, guilt or uncertainty, can also interfere.

Consistency is likely to be the cornerstone: reminding the child on every occasion when unacceptable behaviour occurs. The teacher may need to go to additional lengths to demonstrate her approval or disapproval. A simple 'Don't put the crayons in your mouth', may not register with a hearing-impaired child. The teacher may need to gain the child's full attention and eye contact before delivering her message in such a way as to leave no doubt in the child's mind that crayons are not part of the normal nursery diet.

Avoidance is a second rule of thumb. If it is well known that a child is upset by changes in routine, time spent on preparation and explanation can help. One teacher we know devises a daily picture timetable for her children showing the sequence of changes and events during the day. When a child is asked to undress it is easier to explain with the aid of the picture time sheet that it is PE next, rather than a medical examination. When one child we know persistently threw a tantrum for some undisclosed reason every time he saw his mother arrive in the nursery to collect him, fuss was avoided by asking the mother to come a few

Figure 3.2: The Home-School Book

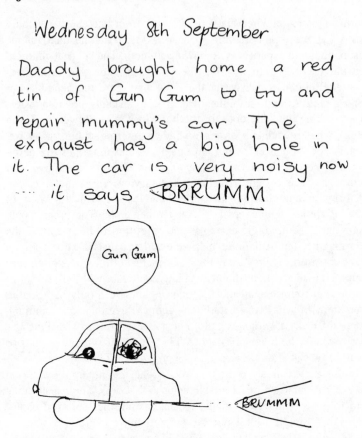

The home-school diary highlights new experiences, vocabulary, important events, and helps the child look forward to future activities.

minutes later than normal and by arranging for him to be handed over at the gate.

A third principle is to be on the lookout for positive behaviour and to be lavish with praise when the child does what is required of him.

Almost every child responds to the pressure of a peer-group situation to fit in and do as the others. If a hearing-impaired child successfully negotiates a few hurdles and learns to conform, this should be given just as generous a reward as negativism requires disapproval. Some of these 'behavioural' principles are pursued in greater depth and in a very entertaining way by Westmacott and Cameron (1981).

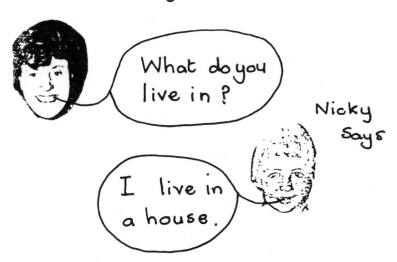

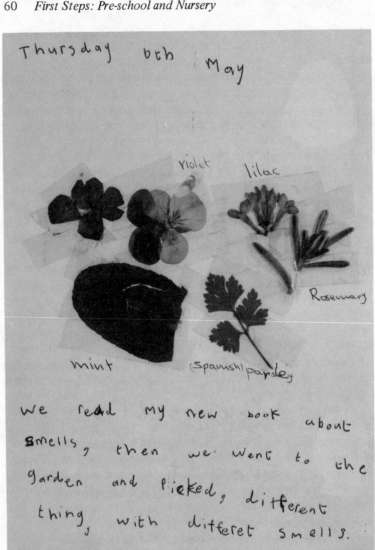

Thursday 6th May

violet   lilac

Rosemary

mint   (Spanish) parsley

We read my new book about smells, then we went to the garden and picked, different thing, with differet smells.

The Home-School Book

Almost every specialist teacher working with hearing-impaired children acknowledges the daily diary which goes back and forth with the child, as being the best home-school link. Young children, particularly those with limited communication skills, find it hard to describe what they do at nursery or school. The parents often have no way of knowing what the child has experienced, talking over and reinforcing any new ideas or concepts, unless there is an ongoing dialogue with the teacher. For very young children spending some time with groups of normally hearing children, the daily diary is still a good way for parents and teachers to keep in touch. The teacher notes down some of the main activities of the day, there may be a drawing or photograph of a special event or trip out, a newly discovered name or important vocabulary. The parents, of course, can do likewise, which enhances the occasions when the hearing-impaired child wishes to talk in class about something which happened at home.

What a lovely idea. We enjoyed looking at the pretty flowers and herbs.

Where are we going soon?

The home-school book can be elaborated into something of a forward-planner to help the child cope with impending hospital appointments, visits to the optician or dentist; or simply to look forward to a holiday, party or Christmas. Some other ideas along these lines are discussed by Bishop and Gregory (1984).

Hearing-aids

The sooner a hearing-impaired child is provided with amplification, the lesser the impact of deafness at source. For the more severely hearing-impaired child the later the diagnosis is made and hearing-aids fitted, the more serious the likely interference in social development, speech and language. In terms of language skills some teachers refer to the child's 'listening age': the length of time a child has been exposed to more meaningful, amplified auditory signals. Hearing-aids will be the least familiar aspect to the non-specialist teacher, but the most important to the child. The teacher will need to know the basic management of an aid if there is a hearing-impaired child in her class.

The idea of a hearing-aid is a simple one: to make sounds loud enough when they reach the eardrum to enable perception even by defective hearing mechanisms. However, hearing-aids cannot *restore* a child's hearing in the way that spectacles might restore a person's vision to normal. In Chapter 2 we saw how a hearing-loss is measured in terms of intensity or loudness, across a wide spectrum of sound frequencies. Most audiograms show an uneven profile of hearing thresholds, with some sound frequencies needing to be amplified larger amounts to reach threshold perception than others, with further discrepancies between the two ears. So there are technical problems in providing hearing-aids which do not distort sound input by amplifying the already better-perceived frequencies greater than others.

The best method of appreciating some of the acoustic difficulties associated with using a hearing-aid, is to wear an aid oneself. Unlike our ears, hearing-aids do not select out of the environment the meaningful sounds we wish to hear. Aids are not tuned into the most relevant sounds, but pick up and amplify every detail in the acoustic environment. The significance of this will be examined in greater detail when we consider the child in the classroom setting.

There are two main types of conventional hearing-aids (as opposed to radio aids which are discussed later) which the ordinary class teacher is likely to come across. Conventional aids have three components: a microphone, which picks up sounds from the air, an amplifier which magnifies the sounds, and a receiver which delivers the sounds to the ear canal. The illustrations (Figures 2.5 and 2.6) show typical examples of the 'body-worn' model and the 'post-aural', or 'behind-the-ear' aid. The post-aural aids are clearly more acceptable cosmetically and are now prescribed for most children, including the very young. For very hearing-handicapped infants the body-worn aid may give a greater output of sound over a wider frequency range. It is also likely to have a greater number of controls to adjust the aid so that the child can make the best use of amplified sound. One reason for the fitting of a body aid to a very young child is so that the controls are in a more manageable position.

The Earmould

It can be seen from the illustrations that amplified sound is delivered from the aid through a tube or receiver to the ear canal. In both types of aid this is via the earmould which attaches to the receiver in a body-worn aid. The earmould is everyone's headache. If it is not a near-perfect fit then the amplified sound can leak out around it, be picked up by the microphone of the aid again, and the result is a very disturbing high-pitch whistle. Not only is it very enervating for people near-by, but it also means the aid's effectiveness is reduced since the incoming signal is likely to be distorted by the feedback whistle. Children need to have new earmoulds made regularly as their ears grow and this varies around intervals of three months. A persistently recurring whistle is a sign that the mould is getting too loose. Many people are nervous at the thought of trying to insert a child's earmould properly. The specialist teacher of the hearing-impaired will demonstrate how the child's aid should be fitted, and this is a small but essential job that anyone can master with practice.

The Settings

The volume and tone settings on the aid are vitally important. A slight change can make a big difference to what the child perceives. The class teacher should know, especially with the younger child, at what volume the aids should be set so that if they are altered by accident or by the child, they can be readjusted. The other settings should not be interfered with and are not, in any case, easily moved. Most commonly these settings are tiny sunken screwheads requiring a jeweller's screwdriver.

The Batteries

Different aids take different batteries, and either the parent or the specialist teacher will supply spare batteries and demonstrate how they are replaced. Some batteries drain slowly, others suddenly lose power. Children should be encouraged to care for their own aids, but in the early years the classteacher will need to make daily checks that aids are functioning, and an easily identified and remedied fault is a dead battery. It is most important that the teacher is vigilant about the proper working of aids. If the child has to cope with amplification of poor quality, intermittent or distorted signals, then he will develop negative associations with the aids and not learn to use them fully.

How Can the Aid be Checked?

There are several day-to-day checks that the teacher can make to see if the aid is working properly. The simplest way is to reduce the volume control and listen to the output, which should not in fact vary in quality at different volume levels. A post-aural aid can be listened to via a plastic 'stethoscope' adaption, available commercially. If the aid appears not to work the most likely fault lies with the battery, which should be changed, ensuring that the terminals face the right way. The switches and settings should be inspected. The aid must be correctly switched on: some aids have a 'T' (telephone) switch and will not amplify sound if switched to 'T'. The earmould should be examined to see if it is clean and not blocked by wax. The mould (without the aid!) can be washed in warm water. In a post-aural aid, the tube should not be cracked or crimped or contain condensation. With a body-worn aid, check the cord for fraying and the connections to and from the aid. The microphone aperture should also be inspected to make sure it is not covered with paint or food. The specialist teacher may be prepared to leave a spare cord or receiver and these can be replaced in turn. A malfunctioning aid should never just be taken off, put in a drawer and forgotten. The parents and visiting teacher should be alerted as soon as possible. In some cases the hearing-aid department of the local hospital can be contacted directly. If the aid has to be sent away for repair a spare aid should be available in the meantime.

When Should the Aids be Worn?

There are few occasions when the child needs to take his hearing-aids off. Some vigorous physical games might result in cords being pulled loose, and aids are not designed to function underwater. Several children we know have forgotten to remove their aids when swimming and they are definitely not waterproof! Aids should be worn the whole of the school day and beyond.

Two Ears are Better than One

A common misconception is that children fitted with two hearing-aids are therefore more severely handicapped than a child who wears only one. A child with a significantly different loss in one ear from the other may only wear one aid. If both ears are damaged with little residual hearing in one, then the aid may be worn in the better ear. If there is only a minimal loss in one ear the aid may be worn in the worse ear. Most children are prescribed two hearing-aids because of the listening advantages when the child uses two ears. First, it is much easier to locate where a voice or sound is coming from using two ears. Secondly, with binaural listening it is easier to focus attention on a sound source or speaker and ignore background noise.

Optimum Acoustic Conditions

A child's hearing-aids will have been selected and adjusted to give as good an amplification of sound as possible. Hearing-aids are usually fitted and assessed in very sympathetic acoustic conditions. Unfortunately, the acoustic conditions in which the aids are actually used, such as a playground, classroom or nursery, will be far from sympathetic. It is important that the classteacher knows which situations are helpful to listening, and which create difficulties for the child who is dependent on conventional hearing-aids.

With conventional aids the child's ability to hear depends on two main factors. First, the distance from the sound source; and secondly, other sounds going on around the child. Most aids are at peak efficiency within 2m (6 ft) of the sound source. If a child is more than 2m away from his nursery teacher then her voice will not be picked up as clearly by the aid. The microphone of the conventional aid will pick up any and every scrap of sound, irrespective of its relevance, and amplify it into the ear. If the unwanted noise is a nearer or louder sound source than the speaker's voice, the aid will not be able to listen *selectively* to what the speaker has to say, although a normal ear has that capacity.

What are the implications of this for the nursery teacher who has a child wearing conventional aids in her class? Obviously, the noisier the environment, the more likely it is that unwanted noise will be amplified to the detriment of the important sounds such as the teacher's voice. Large rooms with hard floors, concrete posts, ceramic tiles, wooden cladding and high ceilings where sound reverberates, therefore prolong the unwanted interference. Speech perception will improve in good listening conditions where floors have carpets or rugs, walls have acoustic tiles, cork or other soft and absorbent materials, ceilings are low, and windows have blinds or curtains.

Classes for young children generally do have quiet carpeted corners for story time and other areas for more boisterous or messy play. The teacher will be alert to the possibility that in the hall or playground; sitting near a well-used store cupboard, door or passage way; or in a room regularly invaded by the noise of aircraft, lorries, pneumatic drills, drumming feet from upstairs and dance music from next door; a child wearing aids is going to have difficulty in focusing on a speech signal. The classroom management of hearing-aids is discussed again in Chapter 4, where we also consider radio-aid systems and how these are able to overcome some of the limitations of traditional hearing-aids.

Integration: Goals, Objectives and Strategies

It cannot be stated too often that children with special needs must never spend time with groups of ordinary children as an end in itself. We have heard some unit teachers announce: 'Now it's time for integration', with very little thought given to the purpose or function of the experience, and consequently little means of evaluating the success of the exercise at the end of the day. Whatever practical arrangements integration entails, it is fundamentally a process through which our educational goals may be reached.

To help clarify our own thinking we have adopted a framework of analysis which can be applied to the teaching of children of all ages. We begin by identifying goals: general statements of what we intend to teach. For the hearing-impaired child in his first years in nursery or infant school, goals will relate closely to language and those areas of development which are intrinsically linked with language. Appropriate goals might include to develop communication, independence in social skills, self-control, emotional maturity and confident relationships with other children and adults.

The next step is to translate general goals into more specific teaching targets or objectives. Objectives should be set down in a precise enough form so that the end products of our teaching are clear. In other words we wish to know the specific skills the child will have acquired. A programme of teaching objectives for a particular nursery age child is given below, following discussions between parents, teacher, speech therapist and psychologist.

Finally, we use the term 'enabling strategies' to refer to points of method or practice: strategies which are particularly helpful in maximising the learning experience for the child, such as paying attention to acoustics or the child's position in relation to the speaker. We take up these issues in greater detail in the final chapter, which discusses the ordinary teacher's role in assessment, planning and evaluation of the child with special needs. There are also several good examples in the literature where attempts have been made to plan appropriate objectives for children within an early language curriculum (Ainscow and Tweddle, 1979; White and East, 1981).

Teaching Programme for a Nursery-age Child

General Goals

Provide play experience which will stimulate language interaction with other children and adults.

Develop listening skills and attention span.

Widen child's receptive vocabulary and understanding of his environment.

Encourage social confidence and communication through gestures, body language, facial expressions.

Foster productive conversation and dialogue through which child experiences different language forms and learns to control more complex sentence structures.

Specific Objectives and Suggested Activities

Child joins in pretend play.

Encourage small group role play in Wendy House containing furniture, kitchen utensils, toy equipment and crockery.

Child vocalises during play.

Provide toy telephones, hand puppets, dolls, toy animals, and encourage pretend dialogues or imitation of what the doll, puppet or animal says.

Child initiates vocal play using large toys.

Demonstrate and accompany activity with commentary: changing doll's nappy, giving bottle, washing face, putting to bed.

Child participates in group-singing.

Gather children in a circle and clap/tap/sing Action Songs (If you're happy and you know it . . .). Encourage child to vocalise and join in. Repeat a rhyme several times and stop at the last rhyming word, reward child for finishing the rhyme.

Child locates a named object and labels a given object.
Begin with objects and toys that the child already plays with. Line up the objects and play a locating/naming game. (What's this? Show me the . . . .)
Introduce new objects in the nursery environment. Extend to names of familiar people using photographs. Naming body parts, clothing, colours, big/little.

Child participates in music and movement.
Play strident and rhythmical marching music to a group. Children march in time, stop when music stops, walk, run or copy a gallop.

Child carries out a sequence of 2 or 3 instructions using speech and gestures.
Use a play sequence: wash dolly's face, put baby to bed. Give instructions: 'Get your coat and put the pram outside'. Play 'Simple Simon says' in small group.
Introduce verbal contrasts such as 'Put the *small* car in the box', old/new, wet/dry, high/little, fat/thin, heavy/light, hot/cold, sharp/blunt, thin/thick, top/bottom, give/take, nasty/nice.

Child indicates his needs through words and gestures.
Use a consistent vocabulary for toilet, drink, coat, playtime, and praise child for vocalising.

Child uses negatives appropriately (no milk, not shopping); prepositions (on the chair, under the bed); possessives (my book, your shoe).
Use small toys or cut out pictures which can illustrate contrasting forms and play a selection game.

Child listens to a familiar story.
Prepare a small group beforehand. Talk about the pictures, highlight names and new vocabulary, cut out other pictures of main characters. Act out the story using toys, puppets, a storyboard. Make sound effects to dramatise the story.

Child responds appropriately to different verbal cues.
Set up small group play with miniature toys such as farmyard, garage, sandpit, space station, fort, doll's house. Give directions such as 'Make the horse run', 'Brush dolly's hair', 'Feed the cows', 'Put petrol in the car'. Reverse roles and ask child to direct.

Enabling Strategies

Give responses not too far apart structurally from child's. (Child has predominantly 2 to 3 word-strings under control.)

Reinforce child's speech with expansions which make clear his meanings.

Example: 'Doggy garden.'
            'Yes, the dog's in the garden.'

Use physical prompts to get the child's attention before introducing a new idea. Try to control noise levels, distance from child's aids and a clear view of the speaker's face, when child has to listen, such as story time.

Use a shared play context to initiate conversation with child, allow child time to respond, don't over-question or control, give personal comments tied to shared experiences.

Can Language be Taught?

We have said that the significant teaching goals for a hearing-impaired child in the early years at school, relate to language. A great deal has been written about the role of the teacher in fostering early language development. At one end of the scale there are some language-delayed children for whom an intensive structured programme of activities is prescribed. The teacher uses highly detailed materials to drill or work on specific points of language which the child appears unable to acquire spontaneously. At the other end of the scale some researchers such as Tough (1973) argue that the good nursery provides a rich experience which stimulates the child's interest, excitement and initial response. The good teacher elaborates and expands upon what the child initiates through the opportunities which arise for adult-child exchanges.

We would not advocate to the ordinary teachers who come into contact with hearing-impaired children that they should work on language structures in a programmed way, although this kind of systematic teaching of language might be appropriate in another context (see Figure 3.3). There are in any case practical limitations to the amount of time that can be spent with any individual child in the way that a speech therapist might. A review of 24 language-training programmes which focus on the early production and comprehension of specific

Figure 3.3: Intensive Auditory Training with a Specialist Teacher

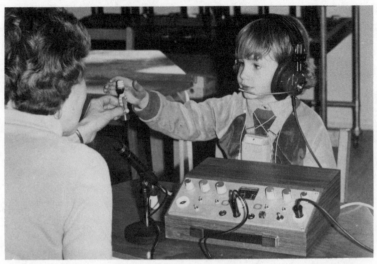

The specialist teacher gives this child an individual 'speech and language' session using an auditory trainer, which gives high-quality sound input across a broad range of frequencies.

features of spoken language is given by Harris (1984). He shares the view expressed here that language cannot be dispensed bit by bit from a teaching package. There must be a greater understanding of the social-interactive and cognitive foundations for language growth, as well as an awareness that in the appropriate environment, children make an important contribution to developing their own linguistic skills.

We would argue then, as others have (Wells, 1979), that children learn language through their linguistic interactions with others. It is therefore, the quality of such interactions that we draw attention to, as the most effective teaching tool. It is important that teachers consider carefully the language goals and specific objectives for a particular child, together with the linguistic experiences through which they may be reached.

Lessons from Mother/Baby Talk

In general, what is likely to benefit the hearing-impaired child in terms of fostering language development is also likely to be good practice for all children at this early stage. We know from work such as by Snow and Ferguson (1977) that children learn through patterns of verbal interaction which develop with adult caretakers. The following 'conversation' was recorded between a normal two-year-old and her mother:

Child: Lizzie car.
Adult: No, Lizzie's not going in the car.
Child: Mummy car.
Adult: No, I'm staying here with you.
Child: Daddy car.
Adult: Yes, Daddy's gone to work in the car.

Most adults make a range of adjustments when talking to children with emerging language, which suggests some intuitive function. This parent expands the child's utterance, restating what the child has said in a fuller way, bringing in additional information, as well as interpreting and making explicit the child's meaning. The child is not overwhelmed by a barrage of conversation since the adult tunes her own sentence complexity appropriately to the child's own. The child takes an active part. We can describe this very simple exchange as a 'conversation' because the vital ingredient is that the child and the adult are focusing their minds upon the same topic (Brown, 1977) and both are trying to understand and be understood. There are good reasons to suggest that adults who use strategies such as expansion and paraphrase do help young children to make progress and there are obviously lessons to be learnt from how mothers naturally talk to their children.

Conversation Styles

It may be more difficult to make intuitive adjustments to the kind of sentences we use with older hearing-impaired children who may still be at a one to two-word-string level. We do know that at whatever level the child is linguistically, the quality of verbal interaction depends also on the teacher's individual style. In a recent study of pre-school children in playgroups and nurseries, Wood, McMahon and Cranstoun (1980) have looked in some detail at the way in which adults behave and the effects this has on productive language exchanges between adult and child. Some of Wood's nursery staff behaved as managers, and verbal exchanges with children reflected a concern to organise resources efficiently, ensure children were in the right place with the right materials, and generally make the day run smoothly:

Child: I've finished my painting now.
Adult: Oh, that's nice. Go and put it near your peg — go on, good
          boy. Jilly, I hope you're going to put that apron on if you
          want to paint. Not so much noise, please, Nigel ... (Wood
          et al. 1980, p. 12)

In this extract the adult does not take up the opportunity offered by
the child at the beginning to enter into an exchange about the child's
work and to share in the child's interest. This adult is poor at fostering
the kind of dialogue to which both child and adult contribute ideas
which linguists feel is important for language growth, although this
adult may well be a very good organiser.

Focusing specifically on what fostered sustained verbal interactions
between adult and child, the least effective of Wood's nursery staff
were those who controlled conversations by asking many questions,
particularly open questions (What did we do yesterday?) or questions
which test the child (What colour is your jumper?). Similarly, teachers
who used enforced repetition (We should say 'I bought a lolly', not 'I
buyed'), or who asked the child to repeat a sentence (What did you
say?), were unlikely to foster productive dialogue. On the other hand,
some staff showed a much more genuine interest in the child's own
experiences, what he had to say about his family or pets, and opportunities for talk were taken up relating closely to the child's own play.
The child would contribute more when the adult made comments of a
personal kind ('I used to like going to the circus'), but tied closely to a
shared recent or current experience. Similarly, adults who listened carefully to what the child had to say, who handed the conversation back
to the child each time and who waited for the child to reply, enjoyed
much more fulfilling exchanges with the children in their care.

Most nursery school environments put a lot of emphasis on providing and creating opportunities for imaginative play. When children need
a little help to get started, books, displays, nature corners and pictures
can be a shared experience around which conversation arises. A doll's
house, farmyard, garage, sand pit, fort or Wendy House, all provide an
immediate play context which can stimulate verbal interchange
between adult and child, or child and child:

Child: He got run over.
Adult: It looks like a bus.
Child: No, a lorry. A policeman's coming.
Adult: I'll bet he was hurt.
Child: Take him to hospital.

In this extract both the child and the teacher are giving a commentary on the child's activity. The teacher's input helps to move the child on in his thinking without controlling or directing the play.

The Importance of Play

It is worth thinking in some detail about shared play in the nursery because the hearing-impaired child often starts out at a disadvantage. He may be wary of new situations and new materials; he may want to hold tightly to toys because of inexperience in sharing. Where communication has made explanation difficult, a child may find himself unable to wait, to take turns or to sustain his attention. His first reaction may be to stand on the periphery and observe.

Other children at play do provide models of social behaviour as well as sources of language stimulation and interaction at the child's interest level. Most nurseries have materials and equipment which the child will not have met before and which the child can discover and enjoy. But it is the subtlety of the contributions which adults make to play which either encourages or discourages the child.

Some of these issues were addressed recently in a Schools Council Project which had the specific objective of studying ways in which play can be structured in infant classes to make it a learning process (Manning and Sharp, 1977). One point which is made strongly is that setting out a rich array of materials and activities which children can choose for themselves, is insufficient. Hearing-impaired children, particularly, may be overwhelmed by the presentation of too many new options. The skilled teacher is not just a provider of resources. Far more important aspects of the teacher's role in structuring play, concern the way in which the adult participates in the child's experience, how the adult initiates *new* experience, and when it seems appropriate to make more active intervention in play. The Schools Council Project suggests that adults participate most effectively by sharing, or even playing alongside children, without directing or dominating. A good teacher is able to point the child's enquiry by suggesting new possibilities, material, information or ideas, which enable a play situation to be developed or extended. If the play is being disrupted by a child, where there may be danger or misuse of materials, or when a problem needs to be solved or brought to a logical solution, then the skilled teacher is sensitive to the need for more positive direction and control.

With hearing-impaired children the teacher may have to develop some initial strategies for involving the child in play. An effective way of arousing a child's interest is for the adult simply to go ahead and get on with a task in proximity to the child. Most children will investigate what it is that seems to be capturing the interest of the adult and will want to join in. One useful ploy which teachers sometimes use with hearing-impaired children is the making of deliberate mistakes. An adult who makes silly mistakes can catch an inhibited child unawares and surprise him in to joining in. This is also useful in checking that the child understands the play context. Counting items wrongly, laying out the Wendy House 'place-settings' incorrectly, fitting a toy together the wrong way round or misplacing a piece in a puzzle, may well tempt a child to join in and put the adult right.

Manning and Sharp (1977), which summarises the Schools Council Project, is a very useful source book of ideas as to how play situations can be created, and includes sections on domestic play; using materials to construct things; make-believe play such as dressing up; play with natural materials such as sand, shells, wood, together with outdoor play. At each point teachers are asked to examine what it is that a play experience might achieve for a child, where the teacher can bring out further possibilities in the play, and how and why the teacher can get involved. There is also a very salutory allusion to the dangers of over-interference through what is known as the 'grandparent syndrome': 'too many suggestions and ideas . . . too much joining in, too much encouragement' (Manning and Sharp 1977, p. 27).

In summary, there is a consensus of agreement in the literature that play experience, particularly representational play which involves the child in an imaginary context, is a foundation to the child's understanding and broader intellectual use of symbols (Cooper, Moodley and Reynell, 1978). Meaningful play developmentally presages and is enmeshed with the comprehension of language and the use of language in thinking. At the end of this chapter we have given a selection of play activities which can be used with the hearing-impaired child in an ordinary group, and which directly help the child's receptivity to language.

What Does the Teacher Need to do Differently?

Teachers are often concerned about the things which they need to do specially or differently in their interactions with hearing-impaired children. There will indeed be situations which arise with children whose communication skills are poor, when the usual strategies in conversation, for example, will need to be modified. We have, up to this point, discussed some of the broad principles involved in play, in fostering language, in dialogue and in styles of adult/child talk. We have highlighted some of the recent research with normally hearing children which shows, for example, that when adults give personal contributions, use phatics ('Ooh, that's nice'), and do not over-question, this is more likely to stimulate spontaneous contributions from the children themselves.

In fact, the same broad principles which are effective for normal children are also the most appropriate to apply to the hearing-impaired. What is true, as a recent article by Wood and Wood (1984) illustrates, is that when teachers talk to the severely hearing-impaired, there will be more confusions and misunderstandings which lead to more questioning styles and requests for repetition, with fewer personal contributions and less productive interaction. In other words, we need to be acutely aware of what *not* to do less effectively with the hearing-impaired than we do with normally hearing children! There are, however, some less daunting practical suggestions which the non-specialist teacher can keep at hand!

Gaining the Child's Attention

We sometimes assume that if a teacher speaks to a normal child, the child will listen and respond appropriately, even though he might be engaged in something else. Children seem to develop a kind of multi-channel attention. They can see, feel and hear things all at the same time. However, hearing-impaired children have great difficulty listening whilst looking at something else. So the first step is to get the child's attention. It is pointless to give an instruction before being sure the child's attention is caught, although one might do exactly that with a normally hearing child. Eye-contact for an older child, a nudge, or perhaps a touch on the elbow, or calling the child's name, will signal that attention is required and the child will look at the speaker's face so that none of the message is missed. For young children, a face-to-face, eye-level contact is useful, which is why many teachers of the hearing-impaired suffer from housemaid's knee (see Figure 3.4).

Lip-reading

Much more emphasis used to be placed on lip-reading as a help in communication, when hearing-aids were far less proficient than they are today. Children who have the benefit of aids which give a great deal of

Figure 3.4: Helping Communication with a Young Hearing-impaired Child

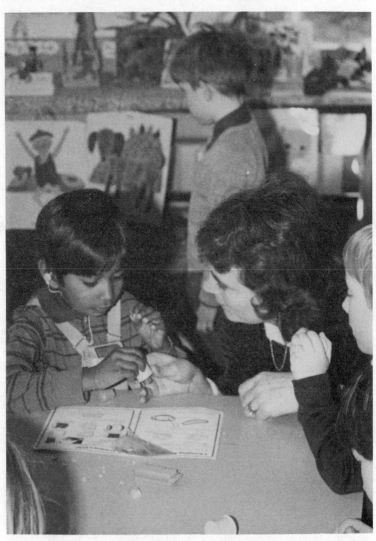

A cotton-reel seeing-and-doing experiment: the teacher checks the child understands the task and presents clear face and lip patterns at the child's height.

useful auditory input will rely less on lip-reading. However, we all use lip-reading to some extent though we are not very aware of it. We have often demonstrated to groups of normally hearing people that as soon as the speaker lowers his voice, mumbles, or is swamped by extraneous noise, then the listener automatically looks up for supportive clues from the speaker's face. Alone, lip-reading is a very inefficient method of understanding speech because so many speech sounds look alike on the lips and others are not visible at all. Sounds such as 'b', 'm' and 'p' have the same lip shape; whilst sounds produced at the back of the mouth, such as 'g', 'h' and 'k' have no visible shape. At best only 25 per cent of speech can be lip-read without confusion. People with a sophisticated mastery of language are better lip-readers than those who have not since knowing the underlying patterns of language helps to predict what a person is going to say. However, lip-reading can be useful as a support to listening. The child needs, therefore, to be able to see the speaker's face. This applies to the teacher, of course, and to other children in the group. Speakers who are more easily lip-read speak clearly, not rapidly and not in an over-laboured way. Shouting, deliberately slowing down the rate of speaking, 'mouthing' and over-articulation of sounds, all distort the usual patterns of the face and lips and make communication more difficult.

Natural Gesture

Normally, all people use gestures, facial expressions, pantomime, body cues and hand signals when they speak. Some people are extremely good at conveying what they mean by non-verbal cues. Take the sentence 'she's having a baby'. A full smile or a raised eyebrow as non-verbal accompaniment can alter the entire import of what is being said. Sometimes when speakers are made aware of their non-verbal behaviour, inhibition sets in. The point is that a hearing-impaired child might gain useful additional information from non-verbal cues to aid comprehension. So, in our view, full use of natural gesture is to be encouraged.

Helping Communication: a Summary for the Nursery Teacher

Check the child's aids are working.
Be aware of acoustic conditions, especially noise interference.
Remember the limitations of conventional aids — such as distance from the speaker.
Shared play provides a good basis for verbal interaction.
Providing stimulating learning experiences is more appropriate than

trying to teach language.
Before speaking gain attention and eye contact.
Use full gestures and non-verbal clues.
Get to know the child's level of language comprehension.
Simple sentences in context are easier to understand.
Avoid shouting; use clear, not rapid speech.
Don't exaggerate lip patterns.
Re-phrase rather than repeat a sentence.
Over-questioning is unproductive.
Personal comments invite the child to contribute.
Try not to control conversation, there should be give and take.
Allow the child time to respond.
Don't correct the child's speech errors.
Don't ask the child to repeat 'model' sentences.
A hearing-impaired child can't be expected to listen for long periods.
Develop good contacts with the families (such as via a home/school book) so that there is carry-over of language experience.

Postscript: Some Listening Games

Some of the teachers we have worked with have wanted to include a hearing-impaired child in group activities which all the children in a nursery class can enjoy and which also develop useful skills. Some ideas for listening games are given below, and more suggestions can be found in the book by Jeffree and McConkey (1983). These activities do demand different levels of auditory awareness, from the gross to the particular, but are not arranged in any sequence.

What do You Hear?

Each child is asked to listen for a minute to identify the sounds that he hears. A variation of this would be to identify near and distant sounds.

Where is It?

With eyes shut each child has to indicate where a selected sound is coming from. The sound could be made by a drum, loud clock, radio, tambourine, tape recorder or other means.

Simon Says

'Simon says . . . ' and the children follow an instruction only when it is prefaced by 'Simon says'. A variation is to introduce an action by either 'do this' or 'do that', where the children must only respond to 'do this'.

Eligibility

'Put your hand up if you have blue shoes, red socks, long hair', etc.

Find Me

A child moves around the room making a noise while the others listen with eyes shut. When he stops they have to point to where they think he is.

Getting Warm

Basically hide-and-seek, except that the teacher makes a sound louder or softer as the child gets near or moves away from the hidden object.

Musical Stops

Children sit down, make statues, dead lions, or pass hats, when the music stops.

What is That?

Sound effects are played on a tape for each child to identify in turn, such as running water, telephone-ring, car horn, kettle, door bell, vacuum cleaner.

Gossip

A message has to be passed from child to child. A variation is to use toy telephones or two-way radio sets.

Buzzers and Bells

A simple rhythm or sequence of different sounds is given by the teacher or a child, to be repeated by another. Can be done with bells, percussion instruments, or just clapping.

Down on the Farm

Write a short story bringing lots of animals into it. The children make the cry of the animal mentioned in the story. 'I went to the farm one day. There was a cow (everyone moos) in the field. A dog (everyone barks) ran up . . .'.

Fly Away Peter

There are many nursery rhymes which can be learnt which have actions to accompany them; some involve finger play: 'Two little dicky birds sitting on a wall', 'Five little mice came out to play'; some require pantomime: 'I can hammer'; some require dancing and singing: 'Ring a ring of roses', 'Here we go round the mulberry bush', 'London bridge is falling down'.

4 THE PRIMARY SCHOOL EXPERIENCE

Our focus in this chapter is on the *process* of helping a hearing-impaired child to function effectively during the time he spends in a normal primary classroom. We have paid particular attention to what non-specialist teachers have a practical need to know, without overwhelming them with requests for radical modifications to teaching styles. One essential aspect is that teachers develop an awareness of when demands on both the child and teacher resources are too great for either to enjoy. The teacher should have sufficient information to organise the classroom experience effectively to include the hearing-impaired child, but not at the expense of the majority.

The amount of contact between teachers and individual children will also vary widely. We have already said that the *degree* of integration achieved is irrelevant to the overall goal of meeting the child's specific educational needs. Just as there is a continuum of special needs which may arise, so too in a good local authority there will be a wide range of teaching arrangements which can be made to meet those needs in a flexible way. Some children will be able to spend long periods without support in class groups, others may need to spend much of their time in specialised provision with only limited periods of integration. Whatever arrangement is made much careful thought will be necessary if it is to work well.

The Importance of Language in School

In recent years primary schools have been asked to reflect upon their priorities in teaching. Government reports such as *A Language for Life* (DES, 1975), and the national primary school survey (DES, 1978), leave little room to doubt the importance which language is accorded in the primary school curriculum. Children use language to shape and extend their play, to create imaginative sequences and enjoy fantasy. It is the vehicle through which needs and wants are conveyed. It enables the child to comment on his experiences, to predict and reflect. Without language, social contacts are difficult to make and sustain. We need language to direct and organise ourselves, to experiment, generalise and connect one idea to another. Verbal reasoning is enmeshed with cogni-

tive growth: we analyse, explain and make judgements through language. In the primary classroom language is the raw material, the
process and the product of learning.

In her work as part of a Schools Council Communication Skills
project, Tough (1977) classified children's use of language as follows:

1. Self-maintaining
2. Directing
3. Reporting on present and past experiences
4. Towards logical reasoning
5. Predicting
6. Projecting
7. Imagining

When we consider the hearing-impaired child it is inevitable that much
of what we have to say concerns language and communication. Participation in the ordinary school curriculum closely corresponds to the
child's functional linguistic growth.

Where are Problems Likely to Arise?

Even very mild hearing-losses are known to affect the child's early
development of language because any restrictions on the child's ability
to listen and hear therefore limit his exposure to normal speech
patterns. For more severely hearing-handicapped children we know
there may be secondary consequences of deafness which interfere with
language growth, such as early social relationships and verbal interactions (Wood, 1982). Consider the number of occasions when children
learn vicariously through overhearing the exchanges between other
children and adults, and the number of instances when language is
experienced in 'over the shoulder' situations. Where children depend for
supportive clues from lip patterns and gestures, it is clear that language
occurring outside of the immediate face-to-face context, will be less
accessible. It is for reasons such as these that teachers often say that
hearing-impaired children need to be taught new information directly,
that large gaps are evident in their general knowledge of the world, and
that far less *incidental* learning takes place.

Vocabulary

One of the ways in which researchers have sought to compare the language development of hearing-impaired with hearing children is through
vocabulary growth. Davis (1974), for example, showed that over a range

of concepts related to space, time, quantity and so on, hearing-impaired children were far less likely to have as broad a grasp of every-day concepts as the normally hearing. Verbal concepts such as 'least', 'equal', 'between', 'always', 'few', 'as many', have no concrete referent, and were particularly confusing to the hearing-impaired sample in the study. The analysis of vocabulary growth in children is fraught with problems, since it is hard to differentiate between words that a child understands, but may not *actively* use. Then again, the majority of common words in English are polysemic and have many senses. So counting the number of separate items a child has in his 'vocabulary' will be less revealing than examining the range and flexibility of a child's use of words (see further discussion in Crystal, 1976).

Some examples from our own experience with hearing-impaired children illustrate that it is precisely this limited flexibility of usage which causes misunderstandings in the classroom. One child had learnt the literal meaning of the word 'time' in the sense of 'What time is it?', or 'Is it time for the taxi?'; but was very confused by expressions such as 'Have a nice time', or 'All in good time'. There may in fact be some 30 or 40 senses in which words such as 'come', 'see', and 'take' have varying nuances of meaning. Hearing children will acquire these exten-sions of usage by hearing the same word used in different contexts. The hearing-impaired child has a much more restricted range of familiar usage.

Some children are totally thrown by metaphoric expressions such as 'he caught a bus', 'he boiled with anger', 'a sharp wind', or 'she didn't have a sausage'. Similarly, a great deal of conversation may consist of local idioms or colloquialisms, which can be in fashion for a short time and leave the hearing-impaired child behind. It should be emphasised that we are not advocating that the teacher should refrain from using whatever language is appropriate to the context. It is a question of being aware of potential problem areas. Where a child learns a limited *literal* sense of verbal concepts, then synonyms can be a source of mis-understanding. For example, in describing something 'big' most chil-dren would be able to select freely from a range including 'huge', 'gigantic', 'mountainous', 'towering', 'overgrown', and 'enormous'. This richness of vocabulary is less likely to be used or understood by some hearing-impaired children.

The language of the classroom can be demanding even at the primary level. The child has to familiarise himself with expressions such as 'Copy out your answers and have them checked', 'Draw a margin, underline the heading and rule off', or, as we overheard one teacher announce: 'I will not have woolly thinkers in my lessons'. Teachers will be aware that particular subject areas, even at the primary level, demand their own specialist vocabulary and language of instruction. Curriculum areas such as science, mathematics, music, art and craft, movement and dance, cookery, games, geography and so on, all develop technical vocabularies and modes of presentation, which may be unfamiliar to a hearing-impaired child.

Syntax

In recent years greater attention has been paid to the child's emerging acquisition of the syntax of his language. Syntax accounts for the way in which words are fitted together in an organised sequence, such as phrase, clause and sentence patterns. Linguists often describe the development of syntax in early childhood by a stage analysis (see Crystal, Fletcher and Garman, 1976). All normal children are felt to pass through the same stages of language growth towards the adult language, although some children will do this more or less quickly than others, and there may be many overlaps between stages. The stages are but a convenient way to describe the particular characteristics associated with a child's language at a particular point in development. At the most primitive stage between about 9 and 18 months of age, most children can be described as using one element sentences, such as 'Mama', 'juice', 'gone', 'dolly'. At the second stage between about 18 and 24 months, children begin to use two elements of structure, such as 'more juice', 'daddy work', 'my dolly', 'big kiss'. At the third stage between about 24 and 30 months, children begin to use three elements of structure in sequence, such as 'Mummy gone car', 'dolly drink juice', 'give Daddy ball'. By the fourth stage, around 2½ to 3 years, children have acquired all the main elements of sentence structure and can use simple clauses, questions and commands, such as 'Daddy gone to work now', 'Where my dolly's shoes gone?'

Stages beyond these levels document the way in which the child learns to connect sentences together and to embed one within another. This is an exciting period of language growth because the child learns how to create extended sentence patterns using devices such as 'and', 'but' and 'because'. By the age of 3 or 4, and well before the child arrives at school, he has mastered the basic patterns of syntax and can generate long and complex sentence sequences.

A very mild degree of hearing-loss may depress the normal rate of language growth (Quigley, 1978). A simplistic view is that the child's linguistic input and experience is reduced at a critical time. As a consequence the rate of progression through the various stages of syntax development is slowed down. For more severely hearing-impaired children complete mastery of syntax may be an impossible task. There have been extensive studies of the range of syntactic structures which severely hearing-impaired children can use and understand (Quigley, Power and Steinkamp, 1977). Most hearing-impaired children are able to understand simple sentence patterns such as 'The boy kissed the girl', and 'The boy ran away'. However, Quigley's work suggests that a more complex sentence such as 'The boy who kissed the girl ran away' would be misunderstood by the majority, even up to the age of 18 or 19 years.

For this more severely handicapped group of children, progression through the early stages of language development may take many years, and it is not unusual for children at secondary school to have functional mastery of syntax at about stage 3 or 4, perhaps less. It is a serious problem when a child is unable to use or receive complex sentences, but one which may not be so evident in social conversation. We have often found that teachers over-estimate the level of comprehension in a hearing-impaired child, and many of the practical strategies to enable communication which we suggest later in this chapter concern the form in which language is presented and how comprehension can be checked. Undoubtedly, the difficulties which hearing-impaired children experience in understanding complex language patterns are crucial in considering academic performance.

Reading

Reading has been described as the 'window into knowledge', and one of the important goals of education is to develop the ability to read. This is as true for normally hearing children as it is for the hearing-impaired. Yet those who work with the hearing-impaired know all too well that the reading skills of children with deafness are often very poor indeed.

There are, of course, many factors associated with poor reading, even in normal children. But a mild loss of a conductive nature may affect reading development (see later discussion), and the literature for more severely impaired children shows a depressingly consistent picture of low reading attainment. Summaries of the effects of deafness on reading skills can be found in Quigley and Kretschmer (1982), and Fundudis *et al.* (1979). A recent survey of all the hearing-impaired school-leavers in this country by Conrad (1979) showed that for those with severe hearing-losses, the average reading age was about 9 years.

Why should this be so? We have the beginnings of an explanation in our discussion of vocabulary and syntax development. For the normally hearing child we take for granted the very rapid growth in vocabulary, complexity of language structure and richness of language experience, well before the child enters school and before reading is ever attempted. A glance at any of the very early books in a typical reading scheme reveals that the beginning reader is immediately exposed to complex sentence structures beyond stage 4. Even so, the ordinary child of 5 has much more sophisticated language under his control than the early texts which he faces, and the sentence patterns he attempts to decode are highly familiar ones. For this child reading is a matter of learning the printed code for the vocabulary and syntax he already knows.

But the hearing-impaired child is in a very different position as a reader. We have already discussed the possibility that he may not have the same breadth or depth of verbal concepts, there may be parts of speech he does not easily recognise, and he may never have been able to experience the 'to and fro' of conversation which leads to a rich experience and understanding of linguistic forms. So the hearing-impaired reader approaches the reading task with two problems. First, he has never met the printed symbols of the written code before. Secondly, he has never met the words and sentence patterns which the code represents. So for many severely hearing-handicapped children learning to read becomes a *language learning* process at the same time.

How to help? It is appropriate here to make some general points about reading. We know that hearing-impaired children with good language and who 'think' in language are more likely to be good readers. So it makes sense to use reading materials written around the child's own experience and to make sure, if possible, that what the child is going to read has been talked about. Some teachers use small groups for topic discussions when attention can be drawn to new language that the children are going to meet in written work. We shall be considering children with milder conductive losses in greater depth, but they are likely to have some difficulty in discriminating speech sounds. So any approach which uses 'phonics' or sound blending may be confusing. As a general rule, whole-word, language-experience-based approaches to reading are favourable, with particular attention paid to vocabulary and syntax. For those with more severe hearing-losses there may be many gaps in the child's functional grasp of language. This may mean that the child will make guesses at what a particular sentence means, from the bits and pieces he can recognise. Children can be taught to improve their guessing skills by the teacher helping the child to use the context within which a sentence appears, picture clues and any other strategies which help make sense of what the child is reading (see discussion of 'Study Skills' in Chapter 5).

A word of caution: almost all of the reading schemes and reading tests used in this country were written for normally hearing children. The sentence patterns used to assess comprehension or to teach reading are often complicated and overwhelm hearing-impaired children. So any attempt to *assess* reading by using a standardised test may give a very unreliable indication of what the child can actually do. Those who work with the hearing-impaired a lot tend to assess a child's reading level by looking at the books and the materials which the child chooses for himself in the classroom and which he can demonstrate that he understands. *How* the child reads is a much more important question than what reading age he has attained. To answer the former we need to pay close attention to the way in which the child utilises the clues available in text, including vocabulary and syntax, to derive meaning.

There is a great deal we have to learn about reading in normal children, let alone in the hearing-impaired. One thing can be said with certainty: for a child learning to read, if the printed words are not in his oral vocabulary and if the written sentence patterns are unfamiliar, it will be doubly difficult for the child to read for meaning, if at all. If we want a hearing-impaired child to understand what is going on in the classroom situation, great care needs to be taken over how materials are prepared, presented and discussed with the child.

Writing

The written language of the hearing-impaired has received more research attention than any other aspect, probably because a written sample is static and less open to ambiguity. Much of this research has been carried out with samples of severely hearing-impaired individuals and we should be careful about over-extending these findings to all hearing-impaired children.

The evidence suggests that more severely hearing-handicapped children make a greater number of grammatical errors in writing, such as omissions of articles, prepositions and verb auxiliaries. They may use sentence forms which to some people seem not to have any grammar at all, and show no awareness of how words are modified in their use with other words. They may use shorter and simpler sentences with little variety, so that a structure is repeated rigidly, such as the simple subject-verb-object pattern. It has also been suggested that the hearing-impaired find it hard to write connected language and approach writing sentence by sentence. The following extract is taken from the writing of a 10-year-old girl with a moderate to servere hearing-loss of about 75 dB:

> The lady carried the lots of foods her basket.
> We went to big park for picnic. The dog play with ball.
> It is lovely weather. Mother feed the baby boy food.

This girl uses sentences of simple structure and which she is unable to connect together through devices such as 'because', 'although', or 'and'. Her control of syntax is inconsistent so that determiners are sometimes used inappropriately: '*The* lots of foods'; at other times omitted altogether: 'to big park'. There are disagreements between subject and verb form: 'the dog play'; and changes in verb tense which interrupt the time sequence.

In terms of a stage analysis of syntax development this child's sentences show none of the complex patterns which allow extended sequences to be generated, and which appear in spoken language in early infancy. Since there are many errors, omissions and unusual usages in the writings of hearing-impaired children, some authors describe such language as being immature and also deviant. For further discussions on written language in the hearing-impaired see Quigley and Kretschmer (1982).

We have to look once again to the problems which hearing-impaired children experience in mastering the linguistic system, to account for some of the features which appear in writing. It is probably true that hearing-impaired children do acquire linguistic rules, but this takes a very much longer time, and the more severely handicapped the child, the greater the gap between himself and his peers. It is also worth noting that an older hearing-impaired child may be attempting to use his limited language to express fairly sophisticated ideas and concepts. His written language may look odd or deviant because his primitive language system breaks down under the pressure of his communication needs. He may be trying to convey a complex message, without the means to do so. It is quite unfair to such a child then, to judge his level of understanding and the quality of his ideas, by what he can put down grammatically on paper.

Mathematics

$$2 \in \{2, 4, 6, 8\}$$
$$6 \in \{2, 4, 6, 8\}$$
$$7 \notin \{2, 4, 6, 8\}$$

It could be argued that the mathematical statements above require little explication because the meaning of the symbols emerges through contrast and needs no verbal gloss. A recent study by Wood, Wood and Howarth (1983) shows that severely hearing-impaired children are able to acquire the concepts of mathematics in the same way as hearing children, although they may be delayed in their attainment.

When teachers present mathematical notation to children in primary schools, attempts are usually made to relate process or symbol to the child's everyday experience. The concept of 'being a member of' in relation to the number sets above, would no doubt be illustrated with verbal examples. The point to be made then, is that the logic of mathematics *is* open to the hearing-impaired. But the language of instruction may limit the rate of progress. This is particularly true when a child has to listen to lengthy explanations with little concrete experience. When new and fairly specialised terminology is introduced (multiplication, partition of sets, quadrilateral, symmetry, remainder, equivalence) great care will need to be taken that the hearing-impaired child has more chance to hear and use these words. So too the written language of many early maths books is much more demanding to the hearing-impaired child than the level of mathematics presented. A simple arithmetic task, such as 'If 3 boys had 15p which was divided equally among themselves, how much would each boy receive?', assumes a fairly complex linguistic dimension.

Fortunately, it is possible in the early stages of mathematical teaching to interrelate formal process with concrete experience. Almost all of the basic arithmetic operations, together with skill areas such as time, money and measurement, can be introduced through real-life 'doing' and 'seeing' experiences.

Other Areas of the Curriculum

Many of the points we have made about core subjects like reading and mathematics, apply equally to other areas of the curriculum. Where children may need to spend long periods listening, and where there is a sizeable linguistic and formal content, then the hearing-impaired child's participation in ordinary teaching groups may be more restricted. Parts of the curriculum with less academic and verbal content such as games, PE, dance, drama, craft, art, pottery, are more likely to be open to more severely hearing-impaired children with less detailed preparation required.

It is important to clarify which aspects of the total school curriculum the special needs child is going to have access to. Whilst specialist staff are often involved in planning appropriate curricular needs, it should be a joint responsibility which includes staff from the main body of the school to discuss which aspects of the curriculum are made available and how this is to be achieved. It must always be remembered that the obstacles to learning for the hearing-impaired child are not related to ability, but to the range, depth, mode and amount of language involved: how information is given out, recorded, reinforced, and tied in with the rest of his learning experience.

Goals, Objectives and Strategies

We have throughout this book, adopted a consistent method of examining the teaching curriculum for hearing-impaired children of all ages in the ordinary school. We begin with goals. We might start out with some general statements such as aiming to prepare a child to use his resources to the full; to develop as a person, socially and emotionally; to be able to make rewarding relationships; to enjoy and understand other people; to have respect and consideration; to function effectively in school, at home or at work.

These general goals in themselves are not very specific, although as we have seen, they are closely associated with deep moral and social issues and continue to occupy a lot of people's thinking. In fact we might forgive a teacher for not knowing when these goals had been reached by a particular child, despite their importance. We shall argue that teachers can help themselves and their children by paying much closer attention to the *content* of the curriculum. Working amongst children with global learning difficulties, Ainscow and Tweddle (1979) argue strongly that effective teaching begins with a clear statement of intentions: what areas of learning, in terms of specific skills or content, the child should have mastered in the teaching process.

Finally, having decided *what* to teach, thought needs to be given to teaching method. In fact the Warnock Report (1978) suggests that there has been 'too much preoccupation' with teaching method in educational research. It is our own view that it would place too great a demand on teachers to change drastically their teaching methods. We prefer the term 'enabling strategies' to refer to the ways in which the classroom experience can be maximised for the hearing-impaired child; for example, by enabling him to listen more effectively in poor acoustic conditions through a radio aid.

The Importance of Objectives

Many teachers think carefully about their aims and methods but ignore content. It is easy to understand why. Detailed forward planning of materials, the information areas to be covered, what the teacher hopes to do in an area of the curriculum and what skills and knowledge he hopes the child will have acquired by the end of the lesson/week/ month/term, are all time-consuming exercises.

There are good reasons why it would be helpful to get down to this level of curricular planning, if only in specific areas of the timetable and for specific children. In many instances there will be more than one teacher working with the hearing-impaired child, even in the infant school. A child may spend only part of his day in mainstream groups, whilst the rest of the time is spent in a unit with the specialist teacher. Or a visiting teacher may support the child on a weekly basis, perhaps withdrawing the child, or working individually in the classroom. It is crucial in such situations, that the teachers know what the child has been doing so that they can work together. And of course the responsibility for what is taught in a mainstream class must lie with the ordinary teacher.

Forward planning of lesson content would help the decision-making process when a child's timetable is devised. Which lessons would be more meaningful to a hearing-impaired child who finds abstract concepts difficult to acquire? Which lessons have more 'doing' and visual content? Is there a lot of new vocabulary, and unfamiliar terminology, such as some science areas? Will the child be meeting new ways of presenting material such as graphs or block tables? Will the lesson have a lot of information and factual content? Will there be copying from books or blackboard? What will the child have to listen to, read, or work on for himself? The well-prepared teacher who can articulate what he is going to cover in his teaching can give a very valuable contribution to the discussions which must take place for every special needs child regarding which parts of the ordinary school curriculum an individual is going to have access to.

Co-ordinating Work Between Unit and Mainstream

If the teacher's lesson objectives are clearly stated and the content prepared in advance, there will be time for any supportive work by a unit teacher or the like, to prepare the child in advance. It may be that some content areas will be too demanding and the range of subjects the child can cope with needs to be reduced in co-ordination with any extra help available. Where the child is going to participate, any new, specialist or technical vocabulary can be gone over. The hearing-impaired child would have the advantage over his peers that he is not meeting new concepts absolutely fresh, and perhaps will be able to keep pace, should he miss a nuance or misunderstand some of what is said. With a carefully prepared knowledge base of what he is about to receive, the child is much more likely to follow, comprehend and learn from his integrated experience.

Furthermore, at the end of the lesson, other work can be geared to reinforcing the content covered. It is much easier to check on what the child has actually taken in and understood if there are clear reference points. Using clearly stated objectives as a baseline it is much easier to make a realistic appraisal of the child's progress, where subject difficulties are arising, what further help needs to be given, and where the child's strengths and weaknesses lie *vis-à-vis* his integrated timetable. It is not easy to specify curriculum content, and indeed the kind of detail and analysis required will vary from child to child. There will be many hearing-impaired children who do not require highly detailed work plans, and who would have too much attention drawn to them in an ordinary classroom setting where other children were not given similar programmes. However, it is difficult to imagine an area of the curriculum where some specification of the teaching content would be anything other than useful, although it is immediately apparent that some subject areas are more susceptible to this kind of planning than others.

Working out Objectives

Teaching objectives, for all children, must start from where the children are at. We find out exactly what the child *can* and *cannot* do in terms of the educational skills we think are important. There will be some awareness of the skills which most children begin to acquire at certain stages in their development. There will also be knowledge of the sequence of skill acquisition — what comes next in the order of teaching. The sequencing of learning-steps and the distance between them depends on the child's abilities and speed of learning. What we set the child to do needs to be as precisely stated as possible so that at the end of the day it can be judged whether the child has reached the teaching objectives.

We have given some examples of how objectives can be identified in different teaching areas. These are by no means exhaustive and it is the *form* of analysis which should be noted.

Mathematics

Counts serially up to 20.

Adds and subtracts numbers up to 20.

States the number of items in a set of objects up to 20.

Multiplies and divides two sets of numbers up to 20.

Tells the time when shown the hour, quarter and half-past on a clock face.

Points to odd and even sets of several shown.

Uses 'more', 'extra', 'same', 'less', 'between', 'furthest', 'shortest', 'longest', appropriately in differentiating familiar examples.

Measures and records the length of an object using a ruler.

Shopping games: offers appropriate amounts for items up to £1 and specifies correct change.

Weighs and records the weight of an object using a balance.

Divides a set into fractions of ½, ¼, ⅓.

Sorts a sequence of different size sets into smallest, and serially up to biggest.

Sorts sets of items according to a given property such as 'all yellow', 'round', 'flat', 'smooth', 'square'.

Estimates approximate height, weight, length of different objects using appropriate units.

Uses the four basic arithmetical operations on numbers up to 50, verbally and in written form.

There should be sufficient operational definition of objectives for an independent adult to check the child's achievements.

Reading

Reads aloud a sight vocabulary of ten words.

Builds a sentence from 10 sight words.

Gives names and sounds of individual vowel and consonant sounds.

Identifies the initial, medial or final sound in a given word.

Supplies words which rhyme or belong to the same sound family as a given stimulus.

Identifies one sentence out of three which accompanies a picture.

Points to the word in a sentence which signals subject, 'doing', place or time.

Predicts unfamiliar words in a reading book from context and pictures.

Uses phonic skills to decode unfamiliar words.

Answers questions to demonstrate comprehension of material read.

Re-reads a sentence to correct any oral miscues.

Predicts words of the right grammatical class to fill in gaps in a cloze task.

Extracts specific points of information from a passage, dictionary, timetable, atlas, encyclopedia, diagram, contents page.

Relates the sequence of elements in a story.

No particular philosophy is expounded here, and it is a matter of individual choice what skills are chosen to teach. If a child is a slow learner then the skills may need to be broken down into very finely graded steps with more time spent on each step. The early stages of reading, such as phonic awareness and sight vocabulary, could be given a much more detailed analysis. The point is that whatever skills are attempted, these are readily observed in performance terms.

Listening

There are some teaching objectives which cross subject boundaries but which can be analysed in the same way:

Identifies significant sounds such as the bell.

Watches the teacher when she signals attention.

Sustains listening for more than 3 minutes.

Carries out a one-element instruction without gestures, such as 'Get your reading book'.

Responds appropriately to complex instructions when these are broken down into smaller elements.

Repeats a complex direction.

Responds appropriately to stress or intonation clues which signal a question (This is the best you can do?).

Recalls a sequence of ideas, facts, or short story, accurately.

Recalls information given in poor acoustic conditions, such as assembly hall.

Can give a written summary or make notes on information presented orally.

Asks questions to clarify confusions.

Identifies mood from tone of voice (That's all we need).

Summarises the content of a discussion or conversation between others.

Some activities designed to develop listening skills in primary age children are suggested at the end of this chapter.

Enabling Strategies

Having made the aims of a teaching programme explicit, the hardest part has in a sense, been tackled. We move on to highlight factors in the teacher's classroom practice which can, with only minor adjustments, optimise the child's learning experience.

Hearing-aids in the Classroom

Most hearing-impaired children in normal classes will be wearing hearing-aids, and it is important for the teacher to be aware of the characteristics of the child's aids, and how they can be used most effectively. The way a conventional hearing-aid works, the day-to-day checks that the teacher can make on the aid, and important acoustic considerations, have been described earlier. There are several rules-of-thumb which are worth repeating here. First, with conventional aids the child's ability to hear what is said depends on distance from the speaker, so that if the teacher stands further than 2m (6 ft) away from the child, the teacher's voice will not be picked up as clearly as it would within the distance for peak efficiency. Secondly, traditional aids do not discriminate among the sounds in the environment. The 'cocktail party phenomenon' is a neat way of describing most people's ability to listen to a meaningful conversation in the midst of an overwhelming array of alternative noise. Hearing-aids normally have no such facility. If unwanted noise is a nearer or louder sound source than a speaker's voice, the aid will not be able to listen selectively to what the speaker has to say. If the opportunity arises it is worthwhile for the teacher to listen through an aid to the sorts of extraneous sounds which the microphone picks up. Sounds which we generally do not notice such as turning pages over, crayons being dropped into a box, traffic outside the window, are very disturbing when amplified through a hearing-aid, and drown out relevant sounds. An indication of the likely sound interferences in a classroom can be gained from a simple cassette recorder if the microphone is placed near to the child wearing aids. It too will pick up any and every sound source.

What are the implications for classroom practice? Obviously, standing near to a hearing-impaired child when speaking helps greatly. In most classroom situations the teacher may well be more than a metre or so away from the child, and classrooms are not often silent places. The teacher should be aware therefore of any potential sound interference when the child is listening to what the teacher has to say.

Where to Seat the Child in Class?

Bearing in mind the most effective distance for aid-efficiency, i.e. within 2m (6 ft), a front-of-class position may be no more advantageous than a back row position. In many primary classes too, the teacher moves about freely whilst children are grouped around tables (see Figure 4.1). Another aspect which we shall deal with in greater detail

Figure 4.1: Where to Sit a Hearing-impaired Child in the Classroom?

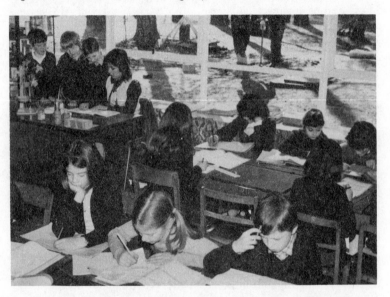

Present-day primary classes are often grouped this way. The hearing-impaired child sits just to the left of the teacher for easy contact, facing into the room away from the light and outside distractions. In this position the child has good access to contributions which other children direct towards the teacher.

is that a hearing-impaired child needs to see the speaker, and if a child is seated at the front, contributions from children behind may well be missed. A few rows back and to the side will generally be best, so long as the child can look towards the speaker, wherever she is. We have seen hearing-impaired children seated at the rear of primary school classes and facing out over the school playing fields: a position guaranteed to distract and isolate.

Some classroom positions will be associated with greater noise-levels than others. If the teacher is aware of potential interference and the limitations of hearing-aids, then a hearing-impaired child will not be seated in a heavy traffic area. Seats near classroom doors, store cupboards, frequently used areas such as a library corner, will need to be avoided. The kinds of unwanted, disruptive noises that become prominent when listening through an aid are surprising: scuffing feet, chairs being moved, sneezes, aeroplanes, lorries going by the window, desk lids dropping, all can interfere badly with what the child really needs to listen to.

Not all of the child's day is spent in one particular classroom. For all of the practical factors which we will be discussing, it is well to be aware that different aspects of the child's school day make different demands. The playground, the library, hall, workshop, laboratory, cricket field, all have different physical characteristics which will affect the responses of a hearing-impaired child depending on hearing-aids for auditory input.

Radio-aid Systems

Radio systems were designed to eliminate some of the problems associated with conventional hearing aids. A microphone and transmitter unit are worn by the speaker, whilst the child wears the radio receiver. The microphone is usually worn close to the speaker's mouth and what the speaker says is picked up by the microphone, converted into a radio signal and transmitted. The child's receiver (not a hearing-aid transducer, which is also called a receiver) is tuned to the transmitting frequency and picks up the radio signal. The child's hearing-aid then amplifies the signal so received. Since what the speaker says is transmitted via radio waves to the child's hearing-aids, the teacher's voice may be heard just as well at distances approaching the length of a football pitch with no reduction in clarity. The position of walls, doors or other objects between speaker and listener has very little effect on the signal. Thus, the problem of distance is effectively eliminated.

Most radio aids now have environmental microphones to pick up sound signals in the child's immediate surroundings, including the child's own voice. This means that the child does not have to rely solely on the transmitter input. In fact, there are several varieties of radio systems, each with its own characteristics, and these have been described more fully in Chapter 2. The most significant aspect of all such systems is the possibility of an uninterrupted signal from the speaker to the listener across gaps of several metres if necessary. The speaker can be sure that what is said will be clearly transmitted to the child, regardless of other interfering sound sources and the general level of the background noise. A word of caution, however: hearing-aids are only one aspect of maximising communication. Proper use of aids has to be combined with many other supports to enable participation in normal classroom experience for a hearing-impaired child. All too often the teacher who puts on a radio-aid microphone can be misled into believing that nothing more need be done to help the child.

Using a Radio-aid in the Class

When the radio-aid is switched on, *all* that is picked up by the radio-aid microphone worn by the speaker is transmitted to the child's ear. Much of what the teacher has to say during a lesson may not be relevant to the child wearing the aid, for example when discussing another child's work. It is important to switch off the microphone in this situation. There is a good long-term reason for this: if the child has a constant sound input of little relevance to himself, he will cease to pay attention after a time. To maximise the listening experience the child needs to hear what is pertinent to him. Those teachers who verbally abuse children for their misdeeds, or who let things slip in the staffroom during break, should ensure they have switched off their radio microphones!

It is also important to remember that it is not exclusively the teacher who needs to be heard clearly. In a small group discussion, or where a child is telling the class about his story or picture, the microphone should be given to the other child to wear. If this is not possible, the teacher may wish to repeat the salient information into the microphone. Similarly, if the radio system cannot be used at all, for example during swimming or PE, the teacher must ensure that the child has heard and understood directions. Some teachers have devised with their children a method of signalling, such as pointing to the receiver, when the system is not working or has inadvertently been switched off. Obviously, there will need to be day-to-day checks that the aid has been 'charged' properly and the settings are correct. The specialist teacher of the hearing-impaired will be the normal source of advice for the proper working of radio aids, and any apparent faults should be dealt with as quickly as possible.

How Important is Lip-reading?

If the child is able to see the speaker's face there may be additional cues in the few speech sound patterns which are visible on the lips, which will support communication. The same can be said of facial expressions and natural gestures which accompany speech. We have so far talked in terms of maximising factors for success. Lip-reading is one factor among many. However, anything which interferes unnecessarily with the child's ability to see the speaker's face clearly minimises any supportive cues that the child might derive from lip-reading.

Speakers who hold their hands, pens, pipes and books in front of their mouths or who have heavy moustaches and beards, may be more difficult to lip-read. Similarly, a speaker who stands in front of a window or light source, silhouetttes himself and makes his face less visible. Speakers who look directly at their audience, as opposed to up at the ceiling or down at the floor, make visual cues possible. Needless to say, a teacher who talks whilst writing on the board cannot be lip-read through the back of his skull; the same applies to a teacher who talks whilst pacing behind his students. Similarly, a teacher cannot be lip-read who talks over a child's shoulder. Lip-reading can only occur successfully in *en face* situations. Anything which interferes with the normal rhythms of speech or the pattern of lip shapes, makes things less easy to understand. Shouting or 'mouthing', for example, both create unusual rhythm or sound patterns in speech.

Teacher Strategies for Communication

The last thing we would want is for teachers to feel that the hearing-impaired child is too special and that the teacher's style of doing things has to be radically changed. However, there are some simple suggestions (which in fact hold for all children) as to how problems of communicating and understanding can be avoided and which are indispensable as enabling strategies.

Attention

We start with gaining the child's attention before delivering the message. With normally hearing children we may give an instruction when the child is already engaged in something else. Attention can be alerted and the message received simultaneously. We expect normally hearing children to listen whilst we write on the board; we give a commentary whilst putting up a picture to look at; we explain a procedure whilst children watch a demonstration or experiment. This is much more difficult for the hearing-impaired child. It is helpful then for the child to be nudged by a neighbour, or to get eye-contact by calling the child's name, to signal the fact that attention is required. Then the message can be given.

Speech Input

It is good practice to speak clearly, not too rapidly or in an over-laboured way. Simple sentences will be more easily taken in than complex, convoluted ones. Where a concept may be difficult to grasp the teacher can paraphrase, simplify, or break down into smaller sets of ideas, what he is trying to get across. Repetition of a sentence which has been misunderstood may be less effective than changing words and sentence patterns.

Open-ended conversation between the child and teacher may pose greater problems for mutual understanding if a hearing-impaired child's speech is not very intelligible. There will aways be the situation where such a child rushes up to a teacher in the playground to say something urgently and for which there is no context at all. We have already given fairly lengthy consideration to aspects which appear to stimulate conversation between children and adults (such as personal contributions from the teacher) whilst some strategies are unproductive (such as questioning). Discussions in Wood *et al.* (1980) regarding teachers' styles and children's conversational responses are relevant to the primary school child with a hearing-impairment.

We are in no sense questioning the value of open-ended, free-ranging and stimulating discussion for children with more sophisticated linguistic skills. But where communication is a problem the teacher will get to know the level of sentence complexity that the child can handle comfortably; be careful about providing a specific context, task or materials, around which discussion can focus; provide a little clarification if need be to help conversation along by drawing a picture or writing a word down; and check frequently with the child whether he has understood.

Strategies for the Group Situation

It is not only the teacher who needs to be aware of the obstacles that deafness may present in the way of normal social interaction and communication, but other children also. A tactful moment or two of preparation may help others to be more sensitive to a hearing-impaired child's special needs. For example, most hearing-impaired children take a greater length of time to comprehend and respond. It can be hard for everyone to remember that the limiting factor is not intelligence or laziness, but language.

In a well-organised situation where a hearing-impaired child joins a group for some but not all lessons, many preparations can be made beforehand. The importance of having clearly specified teaching objectives has already been stated. A coursebook or individual lesson plan can be worked on by the child with his specialist teacher before he joins the group. If the child spends almost all of his time in the group it is still a great help for work to be gone over and reinforced, perhaps by a classroom assistant or another child. For some subjects a preview of the lesson material is essential, particularly if there is specialist vocabulary which the hearing-impaired child will not have met before. Written instructions and summaries of classroom exercises, assignments and ongoing lesson themes, all have their place.

Using Visual Cues

Some teachers have found it useful for other children in their groups as well as a hearing-impaired child, to have multiple ways of presenting important information. Techniques of presentation in a variety of formats are not new to most teachers. Almost all schools have overhead projectors and have access to video recorders and television. Picture illustrations, diagrams, charts, graphs, notes, summaries, lists, are all ways of showing material in a variety of ways which are *visually* accessible to a hearing-impaired child. It is important to remember not to begin talking before the child has had time to look at the material. It may help too, when visual information is being used, such as charts or transparencies, for the teacher to *point* to the specific aspect which illustrates what he is talking about.

Peer-adoption

Many hearing-impaired children can be helped enormously in a normal class group by being 'adopted' by another child. A science teacher was once observed preparing an experiment at the front of a class which included a hearing-impaired child. The majority of the children were so poised to gather round the interesting looking array of bottles and tubes that a simple gasp of 'OK' brought 29 eager faces to the front of the room. The hearing-impaired child was left on his own with his head in a book. An adoptive friend would have been able to 'cue' the child into the lesson change. However achieved, it is important for the hearing-impaired child to be alerted to topic changes, moves of lesson material, any announcements and other important breaks in procedure, so that he is not always out of step with what is going on.

Group Discussions

Group discussions are also moments in classroom experience when hearing-impaired children feel left out. The teacher may well have to make certain additions to normal practice to help the hearing-impaired child participate. It can be very difficult for a hearing-impaired child to know who is speaking to whom. The teacher may wish therefore, to identify the speaker. If the speaker cannot be lip-read, if the child depends on a radio-aid system, or if what is said is too complex for the child to understand, then the teacher will have to step in. The teacher may paraphrase what has been said, illustrate further the content, hand the microphone to the speaker, or simply repeat into the radio-aid microphone. It is inevitable however, that in some situations not everything that goes on in the classroom experience can be understood by the hearing-impaired child. If the child does not have a meaningful experience for the majority of the time we would question the level of support offered and the proportion of time spent with normal class groups.

We often suggest that for discussion work the class is divided into micro-groups of a handful of children. It is much easier for the hearing-impaired child to join in a discussion following a video, radio programme or story when smaller numbers take part. In this kind of situation a group might be asked to devise questions, re-tell a series of events and facts, or find as many adjectives as possible to describe feelings appropriate to the topic. A child may be confident enough to act as spokesperson in the midst of four or five children and the teacher, but feel very exposed and inhibited in reporting to the whole class.

Good Practice and Experiential Learning

For the process of integration to succeed the gap between classroom expectations and a hearing-impaired child's functional ability, levels of achievement and particularly, comprehension of language, should not be overwhelmingly great. The teacher must be aware indeed of every child's limitations in a group if the pace and level of his teaching are to be gauged appropriately. What succeeds with a hearing-impaired child, however, will normally turn out to be good teaching practice for all children. In this respect all children benefit from experiential learning. Teachers who work extensively with the hearing-impaired know that the most effective way to stimulate spontaneous language is to provide a real-life experience. Real-life experiences can be actual visits to factories, shops, farms or the like. But they also include what the Americans call 'hands-on' activities which involve the child directly and actively in the learning process, doing and then talking (see Figure 3.4). Where it is necessary to use abstract or more remote subject matter, these can be brought to life as far as possible by using photographs, concrete examples and the sort of illustrative multi-media methods already mentioned.

The Social Experience for the Hearing-impaired Child

It is important for the ordinary teacher to take careful note of the hearing-impaired child's social participation in the class group. There are measures which the teacher can use to assess the degree of social interaction, based on observation, and these are discussed in Chapter 6. There are also practical ways in which a child can be helped to feel more of an integral part of an ordinary class.

Many hearing-impaired youngsters are sensitive about their own speech and are embarrassed to talk out loud in front of a class. To begin with a teacher may ask such a child to make limited contributions aloud, by asking closed questions, for example. We have already said that it may be easier for a child to participate orally if the group is split up into smaller groups for activities which involve discussion. Likewise, the hearing-impaired child might feel better about being singled out for extra help in class if one or two other ordinary children who could benefit from some extra reinforcement, were also included. Some hearing-impaired children give the impression that they understand what is going on, when in fact they are following other children's lead. Such a child will laugh when the others do, put his hand up and appear to follow directions, simply by imitation. We have observed several children who have kept themselves quietly to themselves, in one case apparently buried in a book which on closer inspection was upside down. The teacher must probe from time to time to check that the child really does know the answer when he puts his hand up, and that he is not copying his neighbour's behaviour or his work.

In the Playground

Possibly the most revealing times to observe the social interaction of a hearing-impaired child with his peers are in the more informal situations in school, such as at playtime or during lunch. It is useful to know how other children approach him, whether they include him in games and choose him as a partner, whether he is invited home to a party, how he is talked to, whether he is laughed at or teased (see Figure 4.2).

Figure 4.2: Social Interaction in the Playground

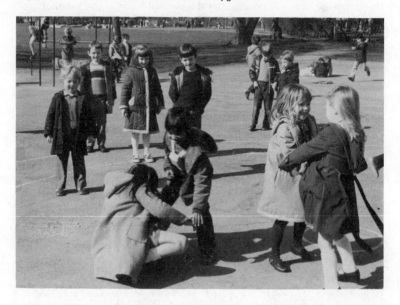

Informal situations in school are very revealing. Is the hearing-impaired child included by others in their play? Do they choose him as a partner? Is he laughed at because he is unusual?

Two things might help here. First, the hearing-impaired child can be encouraged to make appropriate social approaches to other children, and to ask for clarification when he has misunderstood, rather than just opting out of the situation altogether. When children regularly join in with informal periods which are supervised, such as at registration or in post-school clubs, then an adult can be on hand to oil the social wheels. There are likely to be social problems outside of the classroom if the hearing-impaired child only emerges from a special unit to take part in set lessons and has no other presence in the life of the school.

Secondly, other children can be prepared for the problems they might meet in communication with the hearing-impaired child, and how these can be got over. There will be many children who will want to befriend a hearing-impaired child, given the opportunity. This is much more likely to happen in small group activities such as a chess club, pottery group, or stamp club; and much less likely where there are heavy linguistic demands and where the child's disabilities are highlighted.

Conductive Deafness

We have said that an important distinction can be made between conductive hearing-loss and hearing-impairment which is sensori-neural in origin (see Chapter 2). Most of what we have had to say so far concerns children with the more severe kind of deafness which usually arises through some form of permanent damage to the nerves in the inner ear. In conductive deafness problems arise in the outer or middle structures of the ear, affecting the passing or conducting of sound across the middle-ear canal. This kind of deafness can be intermittent, may develop very quickly, does have a significant effect on the child's hearing, behaviour and learning, but can be treated in many cases.

We have dealt with the medical aspects of conductive deafness, its causation, symptoms, diagnosis and treatment, in Chapter 2. It is important that some space is devoted to the educational problems associated with this kind of deafness, for two reasons. First, it has been estimated that some 20 per cent of primary age children may suffer, at some time, from middle-ear troubles (Murphy, 1976). It has also been said that each time a child has a middle-ear infection, predisposes the child to have further middle-ear difficulties. So conductive deafness affects a lot of children in the normal school population at one time or another, and often recurs in the same child. The second important reason for focusing on this condition is that there may well be some long-term effects on the child's performance and behaviour in school which the aware teacher can help to do something about.

Signs of Middle-ear Deafness

Young children in school may not complain of having difficulties in listening. The ordinary class teacher should be alert to the possibility that a child with poor attention, or 'stubborn' behaviour, is actually suffering intermittent hearing-loss. Such children may often be away from school with infections and colds, may seem adenoidal or catarrhal, or be mouthbreathers. Older children may complain of earache, 'popping' ears, or a full feeling in the ear. The hearing may well get worse during and after colds. Children with conductive deafness often feel miserable and bad-tempered, or tire quickly.

There are some very simple signs of a child not hearing well in school. The child may not be able to follow simple requests and ask for much more individual help and explanation than is usual. He may not be 'with it' or daydream during more oral work where children have to listen for protracted periods. He may need to sit nearer the TV or ask for the tape-recorder to be turned up. He may not respond when called from behind. There may be more than the usual number of 'upsets' in class, or some atypical aggression and irritability. The child's speech may be fuzzier than usual, or he may talk softly because his own voice seems louder than other people's. He may produce some very nasal sounds. He may seem unco-ordinated physically for a time. More than likely the child's pace of learning falls away. There can, of course, be many reasons why all of these things arise in certain children. The point is that a concerned teacher can make her worries known to her headteacher, school nurse, school doctor or a visiting specialist teacher for the hearing-impaired, and of course the parents. It is wise to cross off hearing-loss from the list of possible alternatives, as early as can be (see Appendix I).

Practical Steps

For a child with middle-ear deafness, most of what we have had to say about maximising the listening conditions in the classroom apply equally to severe and mild hearing-losses. The teacher will need to think carefully about where the child sits, where any noisy interference comes from, which parts of the school environment pose greater problems than others, how the teacher positions herself when addressing the children.

Even a fairly minor catarrhal deafness interferes with the child's ability to listen and sustain his attention over a long school day. We have suggested that the teacher who speaks clearly, offering a clear view of the face, and using natural rhythms and gesture, enhances how well she is understood. We have also mentioned cueing strategies whereby children known to have listening difficulties are prepared for the delivery of a message. Other useful strategies include writing key vocabulary on the blackboard, using visual supports to oral material, and signalling changes of activity in a very clear way. If a child is hearing speech in a muffled and indistinct way instructions need to be made simple, re-phrasing rather than repetition will help, and the teacher needs to check frequently that the child has understood what he is to do. An important announcement in assembly, a change of routine regarding swimming arrangements, or a request for money and equipment needed in a cookery lesson, can easily be missed by a child with listening difficulties and can generate a lot of confusion and distress. Forethought, simple preparations, checking what the child knows, and writing down instructions, can avoid such problems.

Some Associated Learning Difficulties

We are discovering more about the learning difficulties associated with an intermittent hearing-loss, particularly if this develops over a long period. In early infancy, since the child is not hearing speech sounds clearly, there will be delays in understanding and using language. The picture is complicated because factors which predispose children to repeated attacks of *Otitis media*, such as poor environmental conditions, general ill-health or difficult family circumstances, may also contribute to delays in development.

Some authors suggest that fluctuations in the child's auditory input confuse him at a critical time when he is trying to process the different sound patterns of the language (Downs, 1977). The first three years of life are probably most crucial for language growth, and it has been suggested that middle-ear disorders during this time could lead to a long-term disability in processing speech and language. This would be highlighted in situations where the child is expected to listen for long periods and where there is competing stimuli, such as a busy classroom full of distractions. Whether or not these effects are irreversible, there is a strong association of early middle-ear disease with immature speech sounds, limited vocabulary and sentence structure, poor comprehension of language, difficulties in discriminating and sequencing sounds, and problems in listening (see Webster, Saunders and Bamford, 1984, for a review of this research literature).

For the child in school there are three sources of evidence of the disruptive effects of conductive hearing-losses on academic achievement. The first comes from studies of children known to have an early history of *Otitis media* but no current hearing-loss. The evidence here suggests that such children do less well on tests of verbal skills such as verbal reasoning, grasp of verbal concepts, breadth of vocabulary and auditory processing, such as sound blending. However, these effects are not insurmountable, since groups of children with *Otitis media* who fared badly in comparison with controls were found on re-evaluation several years later to have made up the ground lost (Dalzell and Owrid, 1976).

The second source of evidence comes from the identification of learning difficulties in children with current chronic middle-ear deafness. There seems to be little doubt that an ongoing hearing-loss of only 15 to 20 dB presents a considerable hindrance to learning in school. Lower attainments for this group have been reported in reading, mathematics and general verbal abilities, with many authors pinning the source of learning difficulty on poor listening strategies (Webster *et al.*, 1984).

A third source of evidence arises from studies of children diagnosed as having learning problems, such as those referred to remedial reading centres. A high proportion of these children are often discovered to have signs of middle-ear disease; in fact, upwards of 25 per cent. There is some speculation about why there should be such a high association between reading and hearing difficulties, even for mild hearing-losses. Obviously, if reading is taught in the early stages using a sound or 'phonic' based method, the child with conductive deafness will find a lot of early confusions, particularly in vowel sounds. Recent studies of reading development (Bradley and Bryant, 1978; Bradley, 1980) suggest that children who are good at categorising and recognising sounds become better spellers and readers. Awareness of sounds in words, having an ear for rhymes and alliteration, are important in beginning reading. Defenders of the phonic approach argue that decoding into sounds allows the reader to discover the meaning through hearing the words, and enables the child to tackle visual patterns never met previously.

Auditory factors are important to beginning reading, but they are not the whole explanation. A more satisfactory view is that the reader derives meaning from text by using many information sources: context, syntax, sensible guesswork, picture clues, storyline, likely content, as well as what the letters and sounds provide. So we must keep moderate auditory discrimination difficulties in perspective. For children with poor sound awareness, teaching-approaches to reading should not be rigid, but embrace whole-word, or language-context-based methods. It is a question of using the child's strengths, such as his visual skills, rather than highlighting his weakness, and remembering that poor listening and auditory discrimination are obstacles, not barriers to learning.

If a child's conductive loss is treated carefully, normal hearing can often be restored quickly. It is the unrecognised, untreated or mislabelled problem which can lead to much more serious consequences for the child. The peak of middle-ear disease in children is between the ages of 4 and 7 years, when so many new, exciting and important things are happening to the child, particularly in school. That is why we urge vigilance: a checklist of warning signs and symptoms of a hearing-loss is given in Appendix I.

The Monaural Child

Teachers sometimes ask for advice about children who rely on good hearing in one ear only. The educational problems associated with monaural listening are by no means as severe as those associated with bi-lateral sensori-neural impairments, or with fluctuating conductive losses. However, a few points are worth mentioning for those teachers who are aware of monaural children in their groups.

Permanent damage to the nerve mechanisms of one ear is most frequently acquired as a result of a viral infection during childhood, such as mumps or influenza. A few children are born with an abnormality affecting one ear, such as a congenital closure of the ear canal or absence of ossicles. Very often the condition is not amenable to treatment and hearing-aids are inappropriate. Most children with one good ear seem to cope well in school so long as they are managed appropriately and the good ear is monitored regularly to ensure healthy functioning. The implications of this kind of hearing-loss are more evident in poor acoustic conditions such as a large, noisy, reverberant classroom. The child's listening ability is more likely to be affected by high background-noise levels, and over a distance, the monaural child may be slow to respond and not be clear about what has been said. There will be a loss of directional location which comes from stereoscopic listening, and the child will have a greater need to search visually for a sound source. In a group situation the child may have difficulty in orientating from one speaker to the next. The teacher must allow for the child twisting and turning about in order to focus the 'hearing' ear.

For the majority of children the most important practical help is to sit the child in a position with his good ear towards the source of auditory information. The side of the classroom with the hearing-loss next to the wall, is usually suitable. Almost all of the practical strategies which we have covered in this chapter for children with listening problems, apply to monaural children too. Where children are genuinely under stress from unilateral listening, this will be reflected in poor self-confidence, a fall-off in academic performance, and avoidance of social situations. If there are any concerns about a monaural child, these should be passed on to the support services available to the school, such as the school doctor or a visiting teacher for the hearing-impaired.

Integration Points: a Summary for the Primary Teacher

Discuss with staff which parts of the curriculum a child should have access to and where problems might arise.

Assess the level of a child's language comprehension — vocabulary, syntax, reading and writing may be less sophisticated than the peer group.

Preparation is the key — forward planning of lesson content, concept areas, new vocabulary and technical language.

Specifying teaching objectives helps co-ordination of work between staff and provides reference points against which progress can be measured.

Prepare the peer group where integration takes place.

Check aids and use radio systems properly.

Good acoustic conditions with little noise interference will help listening.

Sit the child in a position where he can see main speakers, give him time to settle in a lesson before involving him.

Attention and eye contact should precede communication.

Use gesture, non-verbal clues, clear lip-patterns, avoid shouting or mouthing.

If a sentence is misunderstood, re-phrase rather than repeat, draw a picture or write words down.

Hands-on, experiential learning is effective.

Small-group discussion work enables participation.

Use cueing-in strategies; highlight new vocabulary, topic changes, key concepts; use lessons plans, written summaries and peer adoption.

Check frequently with the child that he has understood and is not just copying others.

Be aware of social isolation.

Involve the parents — their motivation will pass to the child.

Including the special-needs child in normal classes should not be at the expense of the majority.

Evaluate the child's progress continuously, the level of help offered and the meaningfulness of the experience.

Be vigilant to the unrecognised listening difficulties of other children and take appropriate practical steps.

Postscript: Some Listening Games

Most primary school teachers place listening for meaning high in their educational priorities for *all* children. Using a tape-recorder, for example, removes many of the speaker-cues and demands a focus of attention from the child. We give here some ideas which can be used in groups and which help children extend their auditory memories and interpret what they hear.

Spot the Mistake

A well-known story is read with deliberate mistakes such as a change of name, time, place. Children could be given the written version to check the oral version against.

I Hear Something Beginning With:

A listening version of 'I spy' where each child takes it in turn to guess a sound source given the initial letter.

Word Bingo

Bingo with words instead of numbers. Children cover up the words on printed cards as they hear them read out.

Draw Me

Teacher gives a sequence of directions for each drawing, increasing in complexity. Start with: 'Draw a box with a red ball inside', then 'Draw a ladder with a dog at the bottom, put a yellow cross to the right of the dog and a blue apple in the tree', then 'Draw a house with 3 windows, a brown door with a number 8' . . . and so on.

Going Shopping

Every child is asked in turn to put more items on the end of a shopping list: 'I went to the shop and bought eggs'; 'I went to the shop and bought eggs and milk'; 'I went to . . . '.

Sounds in Words

A sound is introduced followed by a word containing the sound. Children have to say whether the sound is at the beginning, middle or end of the word.

What's Missing?

A series of items is read out, such as names of flowers, colours, toys, places, animals, festival days, vegetables. Each list is given twice with one item missing on the second reading, and the children have to detect which one.

Numbers

Children are given a target: 'I want you to listen for the number which is highest, lowest, odd or nearest to . . . ', and a series is given for each target.

Silly Sentences

With eyes closed children listen to different sentences with a silly mistake to be spotted in one, e.g. 'John put on his shoes then his socks'.

Word Families

Children are asked to put orally given words in sound families (moon, could, soon, wood) and to add more of their own to each group.

Listen for the Words

A passage is read out and one team are asked to listen for names of people, objects or a particular word such as 'and'; the other team listen for names of animals, colours, time-references and numbers.

Rhymes

Children listen to jingles with rhyming words. Occasionally a non-rhyming word is substituted, or a gap is left and a suitable rhyming word must be predicted.

Story-telling

A story is initiated by one child and passed on with every child recalling and then adding on another element. This can be done with a series of simple instructions which the last child has to act upon.

5 SECONDARY EDUCATION AND BEYOND

It is sometimes said that whereas primary schools are interested in children, secondary schools are preoccupied with organisation. That remark is unfair to both sectors since any school which is poorly organised is unlikely to provide an atmosphere in which good relationships are nurtured as part of the learning experience. What it does reflect are the changing demands upon schools, teachers and children at different ends of the system. Secondary schools have many more obstacles to negotiate in sustaining the kind of interpersonal contacts which are an integral part of early education, but that need not imply a decline in commitment to individual children. In this chapter we shall be considering two sets of factors and the different ways in which these interact with hearing-impairment; first, aspects to do with the larger, more complex secondary school and its wider academic opportunities; secondly, issues related to puberty, adolescence and social maturity, which may be more poignant for the hearing-impaired child. It will be our aim to highlight those variables which the non-specialist teacher can hope to control, to suggest ways in which teachers and children can adapt what they do, and to indicate the kind of additional support and help the two may need.

It has been the authors' experience that several hearing-impaired children who have enjoyed an integrated educational programme at the primary level, find the demands of the secondary school to be overwhelming. Yet parents who have been encouraged by the earlier success of the child's placement in an ordinary school, with or without unit support, will be reluctant to accept a segregated special school placement for their child at secondary transfer. These issues need sensitive appraisal and an awareness that it is not necessarily the child's or the school's failure if problems begin to arise.

The Secondary School Experience

There is some apprehension for every child in moving from the high-status top class in a small primary school to the low-prestige, 'new boy' position in a large secondary school community. Normally, children from several feeder schools will come together for the first time, many of whom will be unsure of themselves. This is a time when children will rapidly build friendship groups, and there is the danger that a child's hearing-impairment may be seen as a reason for ostracism from peer groupings. Children who have transferred from a primary school with a unit resource may miss the sense of sanctuary which a unit base provides, unless the secondary school has special resources. Even so, the social demands at this level are much greater since the child comes into contact with many more unfamiliar people and situations.

One of the most striking changes from the child's point of view is that different subjects are taught by different teachers and there are many more kinds of teaching styles, habits and personalities to contend with. This affects communication skills particularly, and the emphasis shifts towards the hearing-impaired child taking a greater responsibility for effective classroom participation than previously. We shall be arguing that throughout secondary schooling, some oversight of the child's educational programme by a sympathetic teacher is necessary as the bare minimum.

The sheer physical and geographical complexity of some secondary schools can be as overwhelming as the social exposure and complexity of the timetable. It becomes the child's responsibility to organise his books and materials, get himself to the right place at the right time, hand in assignments, be aware of announcements, notices, general protocol, sanctions, 'no-go' areas; and all this usually at a further distance away from home than he is used to. A hearing-impairment simply compounds what is already a stressful series of changes. At the same time, secondary education is about providing a wider and deeper curriculum, with opportunities for children to develop academic interests geared to their individual skills. A greater diversity of educational opportunity should, in a good school, imply a greater flexibility in responding to children's needs.

Secondary education has not escaped scrutiny in the last decade; indeed, in some areas the issue of comprehensive reorganisation is still the subject of fierce debate. Curriculum developments, teaching styles and examination procedures are currently being explored, in relation to the underlying function and purpose of secondary education in a society with a diminishing workforce. Schools have been impelled towards greater accountability, and the 1980 Education Act requires much more information about organisation, curriculum and academic achievements of a school, to be available to the community.

There is a much greater awareness than hitherto, of the powerful effects which different schools can have on the behaviour, achievement and social adjustment of their pupils. The study by Rutter, Maughan, Mortimer and Ouston (1979) is important because it demonstrates that variables such as attendance-rate, delinquency, behaviour in school, public examination success, numbers staying on beyond 16, are affected not so much by differences in resources, catchment area or pupil intake, as by the efficiency of the school as an educational community. In other words, as Lindsay (1983) has recently pointed out, we should try to understand the behaviour of adolescents within the context of systems such as the school, rather than simply what the child throws up as difficulties from within himself. Rutter *et al.* (1979) point to the quality of staff relationships, availability of incentives and rewards, learning conditions, involvement of children in taking responsibility, teacher actions in lessons, and flexibility of organisation, as having a salient impact on children in school.

Support Systems and Integration

We have argued throughout this book that we should not be trying to fit children to schools, but working out individual arrangements best fitted to each child. At the secondary level a continuum of provision can be defined within which most hearing-impaired children can be located.

Table 5.1: A Continuum of Provision for Children with Hearing-impairments

1. Unsupported member of mainstream group — occasional visit
2. Weekly support visit from specialist teacher
3. Tutorial support in mainstream — given help in class or withdrawn for extra help by staff member, teacher's assistant, sixth form pupil or specialist teacher
4. Resource unit in ordinary school — reduced curriculum and support for mainstream work
5. Part-time attendance at a special school base with some integrated periods in ordinary school
6. Full-time special school

Such a framework does not address some important questions about the child's experience. Booth (1983) proposes an alternative continuum of integration whereby attention is drawn to the amount of real participation children and parents enjoy in the curriculum. How far do the handicapped join in the social and academic core of the school? Is the curriculum mostly related to achieving examination successes, and does this reflect the capabilities and interests of all the pupils? To what degree does the school take on the responsibility of shaping its curriculum to meet the special needs of children?

When positive responses are given to some of these questions the likelihood of a hearing-impaired child surviving within a particular school is vastly improved. The initial selection of a suitable school where there is no existing support tradition for the hearing-impaired will depend on the enthusiasm of the headteacher and his or her capacity to enlist the goodwill and commitment of teaching staff. The location of the school and its building structure are important factors, for example, in considering acoustic properties. (There is one special school for the hearing-impaired we know built under the flight path of a major airport.) However, the most significant indicators will come from the way in which the school is already responding to children with special needs. Hegarty and Pocklington (1981, 1982) have recently listed what they see as being the salient pointers to good integration practice, such as whether the children eat together, share registration, assembly, breaktimes, after-school clubs, sports, recreational and other interest groups. The point being that integration is much more a question of 'how?' rather than 'where?' this is achieved.

Effective support systems should be unobtrusive and economical in use of resources. Their *raison d'être* is to sustain the child's access to the learning environment without isolating him from peers, and to generate appropriate strategies for managing the child's learning. So that the latter can be achieved it is most likely that a specialist teacher of the hearing-impaired will need to have ongoing contact with the school. A 'named' person should therefore be identified, with whom a visiting specialist can liaise. In resourced schools there will need to be a close dialogue between subject specialists, department heads, and the specialist teacher. In some schools imaginative ways have been found to give children additional tutorial support where staff resources are limited. One comprehensive school we know developed a sixth form club with the idea of helping children in the school with special needs. This was particularly successful with a severely hearing-impaired child who was helped with homework assignments, reading experience and discussion of classwork, by regular tutoring from volunteer sixth formers.

In our experience the most effective support systems for the hearing-impaired evolve in schools which are already committed to meeting the special needs of children with a range of learning difficulties. In such schools the responsibility of providing appropriate course work across the curriculum for the less academic rests with individual departments, and senior staff are involved in the teaching. Individualised learning programmes begin in the mainstream class. The specialist support in the school is enlisted to discuss the appropriateness of a child's programme, the child's specific strengths and weaknesses, where he is likely to run into difficulties, which subject areas are likely to present insurmountable problems (such as foreign languages for a child with limited English structure), how much time needs to be spent in reinforcement work and individual teaching. The specialist teacher will co-ordinate work between support systems and mainstream, reinforce learning in a particular subject, give intensive help in any special areas of difficulty such as English or maths as an adjunct to the mainstream, work alongside the child in mainstream groups and negotiate with others the ongoing evaluation of progress. The use of resource-based approaches to meeting special needs has been discussed at some length in Booth and Potts (1983) and by Jones (1981).

First Contacts with the Secondary School

In just the same way as a pre-schooler needs careful introduction to his first nursery or infant experience, so the approach to secondary transfer can help lay the foundations for success. Since the hearing-impaired child will already be well known to primary school staff there is no reason why his profile of attainment should have to be discovered anew in the secondary school. Well in advance, information should be passed between schools so that an appropriate timetable can be planned.

The parents have an essential role to play in preparing a child to make the bridge between junior and secondary schooling. They will, of course, have been fully involved in the discussions about suitable schools, where resources are located and what alternative opportunities a child has. Unless the parents feel positively towards the educational arrangements made, the child is unlikely to be so enthusiastic or well motivated. Apprehension is almost always relieved (or justified) by personal experience. Parents cannot make informed decisions about a particular school proposal without a visit being made. Usually, transfer of information about children between schools will go hand in hand with a series of introductory visits by parents and child to possible schools. Parents should never feel pressed into accepting a placement, but should share the decision-making process with professionals, and have informed guidance in making their choice.

Where there is mutual agreement about placement some schools offer a gradual orientation programme to special-needs children so that they have an advantage over other new entrants to the school. This might take the form of visits to the resource base to meet other children and staff in the term prior to entry. Special-needs children might be admitted a day before other entrants or in the last week of the old term. This time is used to explore the geographical layout of the school, main teaching blocks, office, library, or sports facilities. There may be an opportunity to experience the routines of registration, break time or lunch arrangements, in advance. A specially prepared booklet or folder with basic information, guidelines, timetable and a map of the school, can be given. Especially helpful for the first week or so of term is the organised adoption of a special child by an older and sympathetic pupil who will be on hand to 'show the ropes'. Finally, many parents are anxious about their own personal contacts with the secondary school and this can be eased by a clear statement of who to call for further information and guidance, with details such as telephone extension numbers and the best times of which day to call.

What Kind of Curriculum?

Curricular planning is intrinsically linked with what we decide to be the important goals of the educational experience for each child. We have applied the same framework of analysis at each level of schooling: identify purpose in terms of general goals; translate goals into more specific teaching objectives; and outline enabling strategies which optimise the learning opportunities in the classroom. We must not neglect the first stage of planning which parts of the common-core curriculum of the school the hearing-impaired child should have access to and why.

Curricular choice will often be determined in practice by linguistic demands: the amount of new and specialised vocabulary encountered; the mode of presentation; how information is to be recorded and then recalled; the language of discussion and analysis. Where children have persistent difficulties in mastering the subtle complexities of their first language, it may be questionable to insist, as some schools do, that all children must then tackle a second or a third language. A hearing-impaired child will be able to take a science option to an examinable level with the appropriate reinforcement and support. But the increased effort involved in absorbing technical language and formal concepts will need to be balanced with other subject choices where there is more doing-and-seeing content. Many hearing-impaired pupils are able to cope very well in options which develop practical or technical skills, such as domestic science, technical drawing, metalwork, woodwork, art and craft, or rural science.

In a school committed to individualised learning and a flexibility of response to the needs of children with learning difficulties, there will be three separate levels of consideration. First, can a child join in a range of core subjects alongside his peers, such as English, maths, humanities, science, PE, sport, art and design subjects? Secondly, are the demands which the different areas of the curriculum make on the child realistic, and where does any specialist input need to be given? The most important question, which should inform the others, we leave till last: Does the child's experience prepare him for life after school?

At the time of writing a high proportion of young school-leavers face unemployment. It is even more important if a child's handicap is going to preclude some employment opportunities to aim to develop a range of skills which have vocational outlets, and to encourage interests which can be pursued in extended leisure time. For the hearing-impaired some of what we teach should aim to promote social skills such as confidence, self-esteem, appropriate attitudes to work, prejudice, sex, and a range of survival strategies. Life-skills cut across subject boundaries, and a typical programme might include experience in form-filling, job application, health awareness, making appointments at the doctor's or dentist's, banks and savings, using public transport, understanding timetables and fares, shopping and budgeting, independent living, gas, electricity, rent, buying a house, hire purchase, pay packets, insurance, and so on. It will be particularly important for a hearing-impaired youngster to be well prepared in the subtle complexities of social relationships, love, marriage, sexual behaviour, contraception, and emotional commitments in family life.

Adolescent Turmoil?

We have so far considered the secondary school experience in terms of the changes in complexity and exposure to the demands of different subjects and teachers within a larger school community. For all children the increase in school pressures occurs at a time when the strong physical and emotional developments of puberty are also experienced. It is important to be aware of the stresses which normal adolescents share and how these may be compounded by deafness. There is sometimes the tendency to forget that it is not deafness which is responsible for every aspect of a child's behaviour, and it may be wise to remember the normal processes of adolescent adjustment in our approach to the hearing-impaired.

Studies of normal adolescence have shifted emphasis over the past few decades. Earlier researchers felt that the biological and psychological aspects of puberty were foremost; subsequently, interest was shown in the social status of adolescents *vis-à-vis* adulthood, which is often characterised by ambiguity of role and expectation. Most recently, studies have brought aspects of historical time into focus. Lindsay (1983), for example, in his study of the problems of adolescents, deals with issues such as work opportunities, relaxed censorship on sexually or violently explicit material, divorce-rates, drug abuse, increased mobility, material affluence, adolescent sub-culture in dress and hair styles, and the social position of young black groups. A major current influence, in Lindsay's terms, is rapid change. He also sees adolescence as being a period when youngsters are receptive to new approaches and can be helped to come to terms with themselves.

In the normal adolescent population there are casualties: youngsters who are acutely self-conscious of their mature bodies, who cannot cope with peer-group influences and parental restrictions, and who exhibit unhappy, anti-social, withdrawing, anxious or acting-out behaviours. Data such as those presented by Rutter, Graham, Chadwick and Yule (1976) suggest that more than 40 per cent of 14-year-olds experience appreciable misery and distress. It is commonplace for youngsters to feel laughed at, looked at or talked about. Alienation from parents is less common, so that youngsters mostly remain influenced by their parents; however, disagreements about clothes, hair and going-out are common. More than 40 per cent of 14-year-old boys reported altercations with parents. The prevalence of psychiatric disorder in adolescence is no higher than at any other age (approximately 10 per cent). However, the pattern of disorder shifts towards increased prevalence of problems such as depression and school refusal. Rutter's study suggests that adolescence is typically a time of 'turmoil', and while we should not exaggerate its difficulties, they should be taken seriously.

Adolescence and Deafness

The hearing-impaired adolescent brings another compounding set of factors into consideration. It is not of course, deafness *per se*, but the indirect effects of deafness which influence social adjustment and emotional development. Most of the research in this area has been carried out with more severely hearing-handicapped children, and one must be cautious about over-extending the findings. However, we have pointed out in earlier chapters that the presence of a hearing-impairment not only interrupts auditory processing, but also dislocates the early patterns of social interaction between the child and his caretakers. In turn, this may lead to hostility, over-protection, fraught relationships, more intrusive and less permissive styles of parenting, lower expectations, and yet heightened direction and increased social control (Quigley and Kretschmer, 1982).

The exact mechanisms are unclear, and it may be that characteristic behaviour styles in the hearing-impaired are a product of different learning experiences and are situation-specific, rather than being part of a unique 'deaf' personality. However, a stereotyped view of hearing-impaired youngsters is that they are more dependent on adults; less likely to take responsibility for their own behaviour and need greater external controls; less well motivated to achieve, to seek information or persist with a task; more egocentric and likely to blame others for their misdeeds; restricted in experience and therefore immature in general awareness; poor at making friends and in understanding others' points of view; and generally impulsive (see summary in Quigley and Kretschmer, 1982).

The most commonly reported view of hearing-impaired youngsters is that they are likely to be much more socially immature than peers, but not necessarily to show a greater incidence of social deviance (Fundudis *et al.*, 1979). The more severe the child's deafness the more likely his peer-contacts will be restricted, the more likely he is to be teased and bullied. We measure social maturity in terms of a child's understanding of his environment, his ability to empathise with others, his ability to temper reactions and behaviour according to situational demands, his independence, self-help and initiative. All of these facets have their roots in early learning experiences and in communication. A child with reduced auditory input will not absorb information so rapidly and may be cut off from some sources of learning, such as overhearing the interactions and discussions of others. Language enables us to construct a framework for learning, for dealing with new concepts and abstract ideas, to relate one construct to the next, and to escape beyond the concrete 'here' and 'now'. We arrive at a reasoned view of events in the world by discussion, listening to opposing arguments, and in the 'to and fro' of conversation. We gauge the reactions of others to what we say and do in a context of linguistic interaction which may be difficult to achieve between hearing and hearing-impaired.

In adolescence a great deal of informal passing of information and attitudes takes place within the peer group. A hearing-impaired youngster may develop some very confused notions, for example, regarding basic sexual information. Parents may have found it very difficult to put sexual matters into a digestible form, and other sources of information may have been only partially or mistakenly sampled. This is also a time when hearing-impaired children may become acutely self-conscious and uncertain about identification with the sub-culture of peers. A youngster's attitude to the facts of his own deafness, to the way he looks and communicates, will relate closely to the way in which he is accepted by others. Poor self-esteem evolves from long-term experiences of failure, or of not understanding or functioning at the same level as peers. Being unable to make friends; join in conversation; follow jokes and repartee; the feeling of being left out of social occasions; missing events transmitted around school by rumour or announcement; and an identification of wearing hearing-aids or attending a resource unit with low status; all these contribute to a poor sense of self-worth. One 14-year-old girl we know reassured staff in school that she was happy, but cried in desperation at home because she felt she had no real friends or the skills to make and keep them. As she asked her mother, 'What do you say after Hello?'

Promoting Social Acceptance

Schools can reduce the impact of deafness on the self-esteem of children in two major ways: first, by more flexible organisation; and secondly, by aiming to teach social skills directly. Hearing-impaired children are often *expected* to be limited in their abilities and achievements because resources for special needs are located within the remedial department and associated with low-status children. It can be important to a hearing-impaired child not to break up any carefully established friendship groups in children transferring from feeder schools. Similarly, where a special-needs child makes friends in a mainstream group it should be feasible to arrange 'reverse' integration, whereby mainstream children work in small groups in the special-resource unit. Preparing children in mainstream classes by giving information about deafness, discussing communication strategies, use of radio aids and problems associated with hearing-impairment, all help avoid stereotyping. A sure sign that a group of hearing-impaired children are suffering from low-esteem stereotyping is a refusal to wear aids, especially the more visible radio aids, and social avoidance of the resource or expected curriculum options for this group. High achievements by hearing-impaired children in sport, art, academic results, or out-of-school pursuits, should be widely recognised within school.

Teachers can build into their teaching programmes some direct attention to social skills. The right approach is perhaps to empathise with the difficulties which deafness brings without allowing it to become an excuse for unacceptable behaviour or performance. There will need to be discussion about peer-group identity and pressure, so that the child can keep pace with some of the current (and more moderate) fashions. Coping strategies can be planned. One severely hearing-impaired lad whose uncontrolled reaction to frustration in the classroom was to hit out at other children and objects (such as windows), was helped by a gradual redirection of his negative feelings, beginning with excusing himself from situations which he could not handle, running off his anger around the perimeter of the sportsfield, and then talking through his reactions with the teacher concerned. Hearing-impaired children may unwittingly have developed behaviour repertoires which alienate them from others, such as producing unwanted breathing noises, or voicing because of lack of auditory feedback; or being insensitive to appropriate moments when a conversation between others can be interrupted. The impact of the child's appearance, personality and behaviour, on others can be explored.

As young adults in school, responsibility for hearing-aids, sitting in appropriate positions for listening, checking work assignments, organising materials and books, bus passes, dinner money, being in the right place at the right time, taking notes home, and looking after personal possessions, should quickly pass to the individuals themselves. It is inevitable, however, that co-operation, motivation and independence will develop hand in hand with confident enjoyment of school. Above all, the child needs realistic and attainable goals in both academic and social spheres.

Counselling Personal Needs: Sex Education

We have said that as a 'bare minimum' children with significant hearing-impairments in secondary schools should be given regular opportunities for contact with a sympathetic member of staff with whom a close 'tutoring' relationship can be made. Our own point of view is that a child's personal needs, should any difficulties arise, are best approached within a systems context, and not simply as the individual's own problem. Some examples of how adolescents can be counselled towards reducing anxiety and social stress are given in Lindsay (1983), who makes the point that we should endeavour to modify aspects of a school's organisation in the first instance, if that in itself can ameliorate problems. But there are several instances when variables outside the school's control such as a bereavement, or marital conflict, badly affect a child's well-being. It may be more than usually difficult for a hearing-impaired child to understand the circumstances and discuss his feelings, and in these instances sensitive counselling from the 'named' tutor is important.

We have drawn special attention to one aspect of social development which may particularly affect young hearing-impaired adolescents in school: a coherent and sensible awareness of sexual maturity. All children learn about sex through observation of men and women in real life and in the media; via informal discussion amongst children themselves; from direct experience and exploration; and by formal teaching from parents or in school. Society's own view of sexuality is inconsistent and conflicting; on the one hand displaying sexual imagery in advertising, but denying young people access to information about contraception, masturbation, homosexuality and sexually transmitted diseases. It is not unusual for girls to begin menstruating without any preparation or advice.

Hearing-impaired adolescents have a special need for help in understanding the basic facts of sexual development. We do not have an adequate language of sexuality, and this too needs discussion in the context of broader societal attitudes to sexual behaviour. Responsible sexual behaviour, its appropriateness in different contexts, and its consequences, should also be broached. A good overview of teaching responsibilities in sex education has been provided by Cox (1983), who suggests that there can be no such thing as no sex education, but there is bad sex education, confusion and ignorance. Materials which deal with issues of family life, contraception, love and marriage, sexual relationships and adult responsibilities have been prepared by Webster and Danks (1978) and Webster (in press) especially for children with limited language and reading skills.

Setting Teaching Objectives: Study Skills

One of the major functions of the 'named' teacher responsible for co-ordinating the educational programme devised for a special-needs child (which is likely to be the specialist teacher in a resourced school), is to collate course plans from the different subject teachers encountered by a particular child. We have spent some time in earlier chapters justifying the practice of specifying information content; what skills and knowledge it is anticipated the child will have absorbed at the end of a teaching unit; how information is to be presented and recorded; whether any special vocabulary or techniques (such as drawing a pie chart) will be required; and all these factors achieve a new prominence when a child participates in several unrelated subject areas in the school. The job of preparing a child in advance, of reinforcing learning later on, and of co-ordinating work between unit and mainstream, depends on the setting of clear teaching objectives across the curriculum. Since the setting of teaching targets is mostly subject specific we have given a well-worked example of how this might be achieved.

Figure 5.1: Extract from a Course Plan Devised for a Mixed-ability History Option, 12 to 13-year-olds

Theme: Norman Conquest

Lesson content: review events following Battle of Hastings; William made the King of England; Saxons fled or had their lands taken away and given to Normans; threat of rebellion against foreign king; order kept by punishing rebels, building castles; feudal system

Presentation: class textbook, strip pictures from Bayeux Tapestry, tree diagram on blackboard to illustrate feudal system

Important vocabulary: rebellion, feudal system, foreigner, motte-and-bailey castles, peasants, nobles, tapestry, knight

Activities: write sentences under each Bayeux Tapestry picture to explain what is happening and colour. Draw tree diagram to show power of king over nobles, knights and peasants. Complete comprehension exercise in text

Homework: copy diagram of castle from textbook, labelling parts of construction such as 'ditch', 'mound', 'courtyard'

At the risk of labouring the point, it is only by a clear definition of curriculum intentions that we can truly evaluate a child's progress in relation to known reference points. There are some teaching objectives which are not subject based, but take the form of strategies for learning. At the secondary level most hearing-impaired children benefit from direct work on what we have called 'Study Skills'.

Figure 5.2: Extract from a Biology Course Plan for 15 to 16-year-olds Sitting Public Examinations

Topic: Plant and animal cells

Information to be covered: definition of cell as building block of life; range and varieties of cells; complex animals and plants which start from single cells; basic structure of cells; how cells feed; how cells grow and reproduce; major differences between plant and animal cells

Technical vocabulary: nucleus, cell wall, membrane, cytoplasm, vacuole, chloroplast, chlorophyll, protoplasm

Activities: 1. Copying diagrams of plant and animal cells from board, labelling major parts, listing and tabling parts and explaining function
2. Mapping exercise joining word to definition, e.g. vacuole → cavity for storing food and water
3. Cloze exercise selecting correct word from list to fill in the gaps, e.g. cell sap may contain _____ , _____ and _____ food, water, sugars, salts, oxygen
4. Comprehension questions in the form:
A cell wall is only present in animal cells
Yes or No
5. Questions requiring more complete response, e.g. What is the purpose of the nucleus of a cell?

Areas to reinforce: understanding of cell function, structure, names of parts. Should be able to draw and label diagrams and discuss mechanisms of growth and development

Listening

At the secondary level it is important to aim for self-management of a child's own listening strategies. Appropriate use of hearing-aids is dealt with separately later in this chapter, but the child will need to take responsibility for ensuring his aids are functional and for determining the best acoustic conditions, with least interference, in classrooms and other teaching areas. The child must be confident enough to point out to the subject teacher when listening conditions are difficult, such as when several people are talking at once. Initially, the 'named' teacher may act on the child's behalf in discussing with different subject teachers how to manage radio aids and other enabling practices which teachers can adopt so that they are easier to lip-read and pay attention to.

Listening is, of course, an integrated sequence of skills involving assessing the relevance of a message; identifying main points and ideas; relating new information to existing knowledge; making judgements about what is said, such as true/false, complete/incomplete, logical/ illogical; and anticipating where a sequence of discussion is going to lead. Active listening is facilitated by prior knowledge. We have found that at the secondary level a great deal of sustained effort is required to enlist the support of different subject teachers in contributing lesson plans and notes of their teaching content. Nevertheless, this remains one of the most significant ways in which any unfamiliar or specialist language can be prepared, and allows the child to take into each subject lesson a knowledge base. There is a much greater likelihood of effective listening over a longer period of time when adequate preparations are made in advance.

Active listening can be practised in various ways. A child can be asked to listen to a tape or story and then to summarise the main points. A series of written sentences can be given to accompany the story, from which the child has to select the most appropriate. The child can be asked to listen out selectively for references to place, time or names in a story presented orally. Similarly, a good exercise is to ask a child to listen out for indications of the speaker's mood, tone of voice, or attributes such as sex and age. Listening to tape recordings is demanding for hearing-impaired youngsters because para-linguistic clues such as gestures are absent. Hence its utility in sharpening a child's focus on spoken content, and in developing critical, hypothesis-testing approaches to listening.

At the secondary level specific listening objectives might be written as follows:

Organises own seating position and aids for optimum listening conditions.

Points out to teacher any listening difficulties such as noise interference from overhead projector.

Sustains attention for most of a lesson.

Can follow the major topic changes using a lesson plan.

Responds appropriately to complex instructions given orally.

Asks for repetition when an instruction has been missed.

Given orally presented information can write down a summary of main points.

Can listen to taped material and answer comprehension questions appropriately.

Recalls the main elements of a dialogue between other people.

Repeats a message taken through hearing only, such as over the telephone.

Makes appropriate judgements about orally given data such as sense/nonsense, humorous/serious, fact/fiction.

Reading for Meaning

When a child is not being asked to listen, much of the work of a secondary school classroom involves digesting information from textbooks. Traditionally, children have to read a passage, to make notes or answer questions, whether orally or silently. One of the points made by the Bullock Report (DES, 1975) was that youngsters were unable to read purposefully in order to summarise, make notes or to follow instructions. Like listening, active reading requires a child to locate main ideas, work out the meaning of words in context, make inferences and develop an awareness of the author's overall intentions. For the hearing-impaired youngster and many others, textbook language is often more complex than the conceptual level of the material it presents and therefore inaccessible. One commonplace response which teachers make is to reduce the amount of text that children have to face, use simplified materials, or substitute other reading work felt to be at a lower developmental level, such as phonic drills.

A different kind of response is advocated here for older children with special needs. Children can be helped towards a more efficient search-for-meaning approach to reading, rather than modifying the materials themselves. A range of techniques has been developed as a result of a Schools Council Project at Nottingham University, collectively called 'Directed Activities Related to Texts' (Lunzer and Gardner, 1979; Davies and Greene, 1982). In general, these aim to direct the attention of the reader to the critical features of texts. In a small discussion-group context children are given various 'finding out' exercises. For example, they may be asked to complete a table of information by using a passage from a textbook, to underline relevant information in different colours, to label a diagram, highlight important vocabulary and ideas, and to generate questions about the text. Some activities involve dissecting text into meaning segments and asking children to sequence these logically, provide summaries for each main idea or theme, classify different pieces of information according to a given schema, or rank a series of facts in order of importance.

Teachers can use some of these principles in other ways. Children can be shown how to use reference books more efficiently, how to locate a topic or name in the index, how to use chapter summaries and headings, and how to skim material to seek out specific content. Children can be helped to find their way about a telephone directory, local newspaper, bus timetable, shopping catalogue or holiday brochure. The whole thrust of this work is towards independence, and using the existing skills of the child more productively to be aware of the multiplicity of cue sources present in reading materials.

We have already discussed in earlier chapters the intractable problems some hearing-impaired children experience in learning to read. At one time this was felt to be due to the obvious obstacles which deafness brings in learning sound-symbol associations, in line with a theory of reading which highlights sub-skills such as phonic awareness as fundamental building blocks (see Conrad, 1979). There is now a growing awareness that for many children, reading cannot be explained as a simple decoding into sound process. For the hearing-impaired child particularly, we have to try to understand reading from the efforts of the reader with his unique grasp of syntax and vocabulary, in making sense of the complexities of the written word.

Until recently most research into reading development of the hearing-impaired was concerned with charting the extent of the deficits: how far behind normal peers hearing-handicapped children appeared to be in reading skills. Researchers like Conrad (1979) refer to a 'plateau of achievement' around a Reading Age of approximately 9 years, beyond which few severely hearing-impaired children ever progress. We have already accounted in some ways for this, in terms of the linguistic demands of text and the fact that for many children learning to read becomes a language-learning process at one and the same time. However, we do not as yet have a test of reading which allows a fair comparison between hearing and hearing-impaired groups. Describing the reading skills of a hearing-impaired adolescent by comparison with a normally hearing 8 or 9-year-old is misleading. What skills the two children have, their linguistic sophistication, and what they are attempting to do with the reading task, are totally different. Those who wish to pursue this line of research further are referred to Webster, Wood and Griffiths (1981). It is on the basis of this work that we feel the problem of reading in deafness should be approached as a hypothesis testing, search for critical features process, using techniques such as DARTS. Specific objectives for older children in reading might be written as follows:

Locates specific details in a passage by skimming, such as where and when an event took place.

Summarises a paragraph appropriately.

Can isolate the main sequence of events in a story and recall them.

Labels a diagram by reference to a text.

Predicts appropriate content when reading unfinished sentences. Completes a 'cloze' reading task with grammatically acceptable words.

Uses context cues to gain meaning.

Makes sensible guesses at unfamiliar vocabulary.

Shows awareness of own reading errors by self-correcting.

Locates information in varied reading tasks such as index, Yellow Pages, dictionary, newspaper.

Makes appropriate judgements about an author's intention to sell, amuse, persuade, criticise.

Organising Written Work

The discipline of learning begins with attention to such details as keeping book covers free from scribbled drawings and presenting work attractively and orderly. Secondary pupils should be aware of the importance of dating work, underlining headings, using margins and ruling off, correct use of capitals, indentation, and how to correct errors neatly. Laying out diagrams attractively, clear headings and labels, can be approached systematically. These are part of the minutiae of self-organisation in planning and presenting school or homework responsibly.

There are some hearing-impaired youngsters, particularly the more heavily handicapped, who are still acquiring very basic grammatical control of spoken and written language. Some examples of typical patterns of writing have been given earlier. At the secondary stage it is possible that a hearing-impaired youngster may be producing written language such as follows:

> The vase is in the flowers. The girl is taking jelly. The lady and eating at the looking the dinner. The milkman writing the book and the cat licking milk the wooden chair.

If we use the kind of stage analysis outlined earlier most of this child's structures are only hesitantly controlled at about Stages 3 or 4. Sentences are not related to one another with cross-reference or links such as 'but' or 'then'; there are many omissions of determiners, prepositions and auxiliary verbs; and the child resorts to juxtaposition in order to extend the sentence material rather than the normal grammatical organisation. We can point to the difficulty this child has in ordering the sequence of language correctly. We can hazard a guess as to what the child is trying to say about this busy kitchen scene. It is clear that the child does have something appropriate to say but is severely hindered by her linguistic difficulties. In this child's case several questions will need to be addressed, including the obvious starting point of whether the child's experience of mainstream is balanced with sufficient supportive help from say, speech therapist, remedial or specialist teacher, when attention can be given to more systematic language teaching. How can this child be helped towards greater control of written syntax?; What kind of language structures can be taught?; And what range of vocabulary would improve the child's usage?

An over-emphasis upon grammatical correctness of written work diminishes the importance of many other aspects of the child's educational experience and may not in any case, be a good index of what the child has actually learned. Similarly, and this applies to children of all ages, language must be learned and generated within a context; it cannot be rehearsed in isolation. The various subject contexts will suggest their own special vocabulary which the child will need to discuss, in order to relate new with existing knowledge. Many children, not necessarily hearing-impaired, continue to have problems in creating spontaneous written language. In practical classroom terms the non-specialist teacher will avoid some of these problems by techniques which reduce linguistic demands. Any written language is more easily understood if it is based on spoken structures. Children more easily write about what they have recently experienced as events, stories or through doing and seeing. Completion techniques provide a child with useful syntactic experience, if discussion of choices is built into the exercise. Children may be given key words to use in a new sentence, or a stem may be provided for completion. Observations can then be made about the constraints on word selections and goodness of fit. In replacement exercises children are given correct sentences, but asked to change a certain element, such as a verb form from past to present, a noun from singular to plural, replace an adjective with a synonym or phrase, or spot changes which have already been made to sentences as deliberate errors. In all of these techniques most of the grammatical material is given to the child, and the child's writing task is one of reorganisation and selection. There are several prepared examples showing how children with limited language skills can be introduced to sophisticated content and given written exercises which encourage syntactic and semantic flexibility, which can be used as a model (see

Webster and Danks, 1978; Webster, in press).
Specific writing objectives might include the following:

Can construct a simple sentence given key vocabulary.
Completes a stem sentence appropriately if given alternative endings.
Chooses the correct word from a passage to fill in the gaps in a sentence.
Transfers sentences used in speech to their written form.
Makes notes from an oral presentation which allow recall of main information points.
Able to rewrite sentences but retain meaning.
Uses complex sentence structures with few errors.
Able to write a sequence of sentences with discourse links.
Expresses own attitudes and feelings independently in writing.
Re-reads own work and self-corrects errors.

Optimising Learning Opportunities in the Secondary Classroom

Whilst we have urged gradual independence and self-direction in learning strategies for the secondary age child, there are several modifications to teaching style which maximise the opportunities for hearing-impaired youngsters to participate in the secondary classroom. We have adhered to the view that functional language growth takes place within a context of interaction and dialogue between child/child and adult/child. In this final section we shall be highlighting manoeuvres which enable older children to enter the communication-mainstream.

Hearing-aids: Personal Systems

A child's hearing-aids remain the most important means of reducing the impact of deafness at source, but care needs to be taken that the aids are functional and used in the best possible acoustic conditions for listening. We have already described the characteristics of conventional hearing-aids, but a few important points will be highlighted again for the older child. The most important factor is that the peak efficiency of the hearing-aid depends on the child being within 2m (6 ft) of the speaker. At distances greater than this a teacher's voice will not be picked up as clearly, and it is quite likely that there will be a nearer, unwanted sound source which the aid will pick up and amplify to occlude the relevant sounds. Some adolescents become self-conscious about wearing hearing-aids and may refuse to wear them, particularly in informal situations. Embarrassment may lead a child to occupy positions at the back or side of a room so that hearing-aids are hidden from view of the peer group, and at the same time out of effective listening range.

The 'named' or specialist teacher has an important counselling role here. At the secondary level it must become the child's own responsibility to wear aids set at the correct volume, with clear tone-tubes and moulds, to replace spent batteries, and take care during sports periods and swimming that the aids are not damaged or mislaid. Similarly, the child must be counselled towards independence in choosing appropriate classroom positions to hear main speakers, and in making known their presence as a student with listening difficulties in the classroom. It is sometimes very hard for such a child to inform the teacher that an instruction was inaudible because of sound interference from an overhead projector, other students talking, a TV programme next door, or a passing vehicle.

It is inevitable that the larger secondary school will have many areas with poor acoustic properties and where there is much more movement of bodies. Whenever the background noise level approaches the intensity of the relevant sound signal, the likelihood of the desired sound being heard is much reduced. For reasons such as this, many hearing-impaired secondary children benefit from using a personal radio-aid system. Indeed, this is an essential facility when most of the teaching is carried out in acoustically untreated rooms, and it is especially useful where children are 'lectured' from the front of a class. A personal radio aid links directly into the child's hearing-aid or through an induction-loop system. Again, the child should take responsibility for introducing the transmitter part of the system to the teacher and showing how it should be worn round the neck. The teacher's voice is picked up by the microphone, converted into an FM signal, and either transmitted through the receiver to the hearing-aid directly, or to a loop attached to the receiver, and recovered by the T-coil facility in the child's aids.

The personal system, like other radio aids, but unlike traditional aids, makes it possible for the child to listen to an uninterrupted speech signal to the limits of his residual auditory capacity. But the system needs to be used properly. It would not be appropriate for the teacher to use the transmitter when giving individual advice to other children in the classroom, if the speech message was irrelevant to the hearing-impaired child. The microphone should also be switched off when the teacher's auditory input would interfere with a hearing-impaired child's conversation with another child or distract him from a task unnecessarily. The most commonplace misuse of the system is forgetting to switch the microphone off when the teacher wishes to have a private conversation with someone else, such as in the staffroom. The principle to remember is that the microphone should be on when the teacher wishes to talk to the hearing-impaired child directly or as a member of the group. Other children in the class can also be asked to present their ideas into the microphone during group work, or the teacher can repeat a child's response for everyone else's benefit including the hearing-impaired child's.

Managing Communication

We mention only briefly here what has been more fully covered in earlier chapters. In larger-group situations it undoubtedly helps the hearing-impaired child to understand a spoken message if he has additional cues from lip patterns, facial expressions and natural gestures, and when speech is delivered clearly, unhurriedly and without unusual emphasis through shouting or mouthing. We have suggested that teachers ensure, prior to topic changes and important points, that a child is listening. Attention control can be gained through alerting-signals, such as calling the child's name, or prefacing a message with 'Now we are going to talk about . . . '. Peer-adoption places the responsibility for alerting listening points, upon a classmate.

It is important to remember that a period of unpunctuated listening, without visual content, practical example or concrete experience, is very tiring for a hearing-impaired child. If the teacher is able to paraphrase and summarise his verbal presentation there is more likelihood of its comprehension. Ideally, lesson plans and notes will have been worked on before the session so that a child with difficulties knows what is likely to come. New concepts can be highlighted during the lesson by writing them on the board, so that the lesson summary, oral discussion and written clues, can be integrated together. To avoid misunderstandings any assignments for class or homework could also be written down. The teacher may feel that periodic checks with the child regarding his understanding of the lesson material and what he is expected to do, are reassuring to all concerned.

A situation which many hearing-impaired adults with good language find difficult is large-group discussion, where it can be hard to identify the speaker, let alone the message. There needs to be awareness of this and opportunity provided for small-group debate. It is important that hearing-impaired youngsters are exposed to the different language forms used in conversation, in relation to a shared, meaningful context. At all levels of development, including the older, but linguistically limited child, language is facilitated by experiencing language use. The teacher who is sensitive to the fact that complex, embedded syntax is beyond the comprehension of an individual, may paraphrase more simply. But it is only through repeated exposure to the changing forms of language in context that children induce the salient rules. And for the older child too, adults who sustain interaction through listening to what the child has to say, expanding his utterance in return, not over-questioning and resisting controlling the dialogue, will foster more productive exchanges.

Finally, since most secondary students will be supported in a tutorial way, any particular problems of vocabulary or usage can be handed over to the support teacher for more specific attention. There are many examples from our own experience, where confusions arise over the polysemic nature of words. We come to know the multiplicity of meanings which different words can have through repeated exposure to different idioms in context. One lad was confused in encountering 'circulation' with reference to newspapers and to blood. The language of the football field ('penalty', 'referee', 'foul', 'hat-trick', 'striker', 'sweeper'); the workshop ('lathe', 'bench', 'chisel', 'template'); the laboratory ('bunsen', 'prism', 'alkali', 'concentrated'), together with every other teaching and social context in school, has its own specific lexicon. Words with multiple, non-literal or metaphorical meanings, are especially problematical and may need much explication, such as 'catch one's breath', 'he was having kittens', 'under the weather', and 'swallowed his pride'.

Examinations

The whole point of an examination is to assess the level of achievement and understanding in a specific subject area. We have already raised a number of questions regarding the assessment of reading, and what conventional tests reveal (or obscure) about a hearing-impaired child's real skills. We can apply similar criticisms to other kinds of examinations where it appears that an exam is not measuring what it purports to. It may be that the hearing-impaired child is so overwhelmed by the mode of presentation that he is denied the opportunity to display his true grasp of a subject area.

It is the language of instruction or direction which often confuses children in the panic stations which accompany examinations. Some specific training can be given in following written directions such as 'underline', 'unscramble', 'rank in order of preference', 'state the relative contributions made by', 'make a list of', 'describe briefly', 'match', 'circle', 'highlight', or 'define'. Hearing-impaired youngsters are just as susceptible to the range of common exam errors, as any other. These include spending too much time on one section at the expense of others, not tackling all the questions, misreading, failing to check over answers for mistakes, setting work out badly, or writing illegibly. It pays dividends to give direct tutoring in revision techniques, making notes, checking recall and practising mock examinations. Some ideas along these lines are given in Hamblin (1981).

Wherever possible, those responsible for setting examinations in school can be asked to consider very carefully the way in which questions are presented, particularly syntax and vocabulary. A specialist teacher should be able to advise on any likely difficulties which may arise for a hearing-impaired child faced with convoluted or unfamiliar language. It is not the intention to make reduced academic demands on the hearing-impaired, but if the purpose of an exam is to assess mathematical or scientific concepts, it is futile to present questions in such a way that the major demands are in fact comprehending the written instruction, the 'carrier' language.

For example, in a Home Economics paper set for 12 to 13-year-olds, this question was given: 'State the different functions of a palette knife and a carving knife, make a drawing of each and describe how you would clean them.' The content of this question could have been examined more straightforwardly as follows:

1. Draw a palette knife.
2. How would you use it?
3. How would you clean it?
4. Draw a carving knife.
5. How would you use it?
6. How would you clean it?

In public examinations care should be taken to select a syllabus or examining board which reflects an enlightened view of the needs of hearing-impaired students. A recent survey by the National Deaf Children's Society (1980) showed that examining boards adopt widely differing practices. Some boards set examinations specifically for the hearing-impaired, or endorse certificates with the fact that a candidate received concessions. Other boards are more clearly concerned to help hearing-impaired students sit examinations on equal terms with peers. This can be achieved by reducing unnecessary communication diffi- culties in examinations with an oral or aural content through aided listening and appropriate conditions for lip-reading, such as correct positioning of the speaker. Similarly, where an examination is designed to assess practical skills, instructions are given in uncomplicated terms. Less helpful perhaps, are extra time allowances or concessions in marking to assess content, rather than grammatical correctness.

Computer-assisted Learning

Before long all secondary schools and most primary schools will have micro-computer resources in the classroom. Some of the advantages of computer-assisted learning have obvious implications for children with special needs. These include a high interest level to sustain motivation, attention and intellectual curiosity, and the possibility of individually

Figure 5.3: Micro-computers in Schools

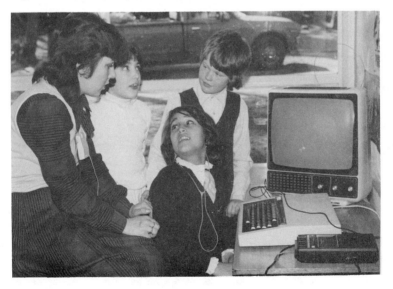

Micro-computers can sustain a high level of curiosity and motivation. This child has two peers to help her but is radio-linked with the teacher. What could have been done differently here; for example, to enable lip-reading?

paced learning steps controlled by the pupil himself. Learning is likely to be more efficient since the child has immediate feedback to his response, experiences a lot of success, and can enter his 'moves' without obstacles to communication. However, micro-computers are not an end in themselves, and need to be used selectively as a supportive resource (see Figure 5.3).

For the specialist teacher of the hearing-impaired there are some interesting devices which offer displays of the sound spectrum to give visual feedback of the speech input. With more general application there are several devices which provide language-enrichment games. These include spelling-correction systems which scan children's work and offer to correct mistakes; a computerised thesaurus which suggests alternative words to those given by the child; and text-editing facilities whereby children can see and amend their sentences before they are printed out. Some programs allow the child to interact with the computer by animating written commands and illustrating concepts. There are several alternative keyboards, some with words, symbols or pictures, which give the child the experience of watching language forms work and interchange, under his control. A useful discussion of the role of micro-computers for children with special needs is given by Hogg (1984).

Further Education

The Warnock Report (1978) draws attention to the transitional period between school and adult life as being potentially one of stress, particularly for children with special needs. There is a serious risk of the concerted efforts made in school to help children develop their full potential, coming to nothing if children are not also supported post-school. It is now widely recognised that learning difficulties often result in immaturities in a wide range of developmental skills which are not resolved by the age of 16. For the hearing-impaired youngster, social, emotional, academic and linguistic skills may be significantly immature in contrast to peers. Many schools recognise this possibility in their curricular planning, and devise coursework designed to encourage social independence and life-skills. The 1981 Education Act also acknowledges the importance of reviewing children's special needs around the age of 14 years in order to plan vocational choices and it is now possible to fund further education options up to the age of 18 years and beyond for the majority of children.

It is important that ordinary school staff do concern themselves in a number of ways with preparing children for leaving school. This must be more than the giving of information about possible career opportunities. Children with special needs, particularly, require realistic counselling about interviews, self-presentation, coping with disappointment and rejection, importance of regular attendance and conscientiousness, and awareness of the increased demands and rigours of employment. In some locations it may not be the expectations of a high proportion of school leavers that they will find employment. Youngsters need realistic guidance about job opportunities *vis-à-vis* their own capabilities. For example, in order to work in a job where there is a lot of contact with the general public, such as in a shop or bank, a hearing-impaired youngster needs good oral-communication skills. Some work situations can be distressing to an individual dependent on hearing-aids; for example, one girl's ambition to become a hairdresser was abandoned because she could not converse with clients over the sound of hairdryers.

Most secondary schools have developed contacts with local industries and organise visits, speakers and work experience for school leavers. For children with special needs this process may need to be extended, and there are a number of ways in which this can be achieved. Where there is post-16 provision in school, suitable vocational or academic programmes can be offered, perhaps linking in with local college provision. Specialist careers officers are employed by most LEAs and know the range of opportunities available locally. A youngster spending some of his time on a technical college course will benefit from the same kind of support system which operated in school, such as prior and subsequent reinforcement of course content by a named tutor who will liaise with college staff.

Where there are no suitable local resources, many hearing-impaired children can benefit from developments which are taking place in the residential centres of excellence, such as the Royal Schools for the Deaf. These are beginning to play an important role, even where pre-16 educational needs have been met satisfactorily close to home. This is a particularly appropriate time for some hearing-impaired youngsters to experience living away from home. Most residential FE courses are specifically geared to encourage social independence as well as vocational preparation.

A growing number of hearing-impaired young people go on to higher education, and some of these are pursuing professional examinations and degree courses alongside hearing students. Carter (1983) has recently published a survey of 132 hearing-handicapped students from Inner London who have pursued some kind of further education in the last decade. His figures show that many more pre-lingually, profoundly impaired youngsters than expected go on to higher education in colleges and polytechnics (32 per cent of his sample). Two-thirds of the sample achieved some recognised qualification. Interestingly, of those students who went on to achieve high academic qualifications (such as a degree), about one-third had attended an ordinary secondary school without a unit, and students who had attended a resourced secondary school were more likely to achieve success at A-level, OND or City and Guilds, than children from special schools for the 'deaf'. It is not intended to level criticism at particular institutions, and the figures are compounded by the fact that children can receive selective education for the hearing-impaired in grammar schools, which account for half of the students who went on to degree or professional level. What these figures seem to reflect is that a high proportion of the successful hearing-impaired children are achieving that success in the community of a hearing school.

A Summary of Good Practice in the Secondary School

Be aware of aspects of the school system which could be modified to promote integration, such as shared registration.

There should be a close dialogue between different subject teachers to plan appropriate programmes.

Evaluate the academic and social demands on each child and whether sufficient tutorial support is being given.

Ensure that a balance is kept between academic and more practical subjects, and that the curriculum is relevant to the child's needs.

Initial introductions to the school are important for the child together with ongoing contacts with parents — secondary changeover is stressful for many children.

Adolescence brings social and emotional problems which deafness compounds — promote social acceptance and self-esteem wherever possible, be alert to immaturity.

Encourage independence in children taking responsibility for hearing-aids, listening positions and organisation of learning.

Take the opportunity to teach study skills in reading, writing and listening, which cut across subject boundaries.

Specify lesson content and course plans in advance; summarise special vocabulary or techniques for prior preparation and subsequent reinforcement.

Within the classroom use radio aids appropriately, reduce noise interference and help the child to participate through small-group work and peer-adoption.

Effective communication strategies include cueing-in for attention; not obscuring lip patterns, facial expressions or gestures; providing a context and concrete experience; writing down key vocabulary and concepts; using summary and paraphrase.

Listening cannot be sustained indefinitely and needs to be punctuated with doing-and-seeing activities.

Language growth must take place within a meaningful context of dialogue and interaction: encourage the child to join in the communication-mainstream.

Prepare well for examinations and the rigours of life after school by setting realistic goals.

Seek advice from the range of support services available, and be totally honest about the child's progress.

6 SPECIAL NEEDS AND THE ORDINARY TEACHER

In this final chapter we give an overview of the responsibilities of the teacher in the ordinary school for children with special needs. It is vital that teachers know something of the broader context of the new developments in special education, as well as some of the 'fine print' aspects, if they are to play a meaningful role.

The majority of the more severely hearing-impaired children we have been talking about in this book will be involved in procedures which stem from the 1981 Education Act. The legislation is intended to protect the interests of children, and it provides a legal framework which reflects a changed emphasis in our view of special needs. At the time of writing the precise implications of the new Act have yet to be worked out in practice, and it has not gone uncriticised. Whatever the eventual impact on special education, the new Act has brought many issues to prominence and debate.

The ordinary classteacher has a major contribution to make to the process of integrating hearing-impaired children in the mainstream. Much of this book has emphasised the importance of careful planning, and it will fall largely to the classteacher in collaboration with support colleagues, to monitor and evaluate the child's learning experience. We will be discussing in some detail several basic frameworks of evaluation at different age levels, and which the teacher can use as a starting point in order to shape her thinking about a particular child's progress. Not least of all, attention is paid to how the teacher communicates her ideas to other colleagues, support staff, other professionals, and of course, parents.

The Warnock Report

The Warnock Committee was set up by the government in 1974 to review the way in which educational provision was made for handicapped children and young people. Its report was published in 1978, and the new legislation stems from this inquiry. Previously, special education had always been defined in terms of a child's handicap or disability. Categories such as ESN(M) were used to label children and determine the kind of provision the child required. Special education in many people's minds was (and still is) synonymous with the 2 per cent of children educated in special schools, units or classes.

The Warnock Report recommended a wider concept of special education. It argued that the aims of education were the same for all children, whatever advantages or disadvantages they had: increasing their understanding of the world, and achieving independence. Some children have many more obstacles to overcome than others in achieving these goals; some may take only a few steps towards them. A special educational need is defined by whatever is essential in helping to overcome the specific difficulties faced by the child in working towards these goals. Educational needs are thought of in terms of a continuum. Any extra help to overcome an educational handicap, could be seen as special education, wherever and however this was provided. The importance of this view of special education is that it moves the focus away from categories of handicap, towards the identification of educational needs. It brings with it the possibility that as many as one in five children might have special needs at some stage in their school careers. The Warnock Committee arrived at this estimate by taking into account statistics from broad epidemiological studies of large populations of children, such as the Isle of Wight survey (Rutter, Tizard and Whitmore, 1970). Whatever the exact figures involved, the recommendation was made that special education should become a much broader and flexible notion, taking many forms to suit individual needs. It embraces many children already within ordinary schools. It advocates that we should no longer differentiate between those children who attend special schools and those who do not. Just as there is a continuum of needs, so there must be a continuum of special provision to meet these needs, whether this be additional teaching help, withdrawal to special classes, or help from a special school.

In the present book we have agreed wholeheartedly in principle with this pressure for flexibility of response to specific children's needs. We are doubtful, as are many others, that the Warnock Report makes any contribution at all, as to how schools themselves can become more effective in helping children with special needs. Whatever broad policies or definitions are adopted, ultimately the quality of a child's education depends on what goes on within the four walls of a classroom. Every teacher has control of several variables which can maximise the learning experience for special children. In the case of the hearing-impaired, we have suggested ways of organising physical variables, curricula, teaching styles and support services, to help negotiate the more obvious obstacles.

The Warnock Report also had much to say about how information was kept and collected for children with special needs so that labels are not used and so that an ongoing picture of the child's developing strengths and weaknesses emerges. Pre-school and post-school experiences are given new prominence for children with special needs. Provision for training courses for students and practising teachers is highlighted, with some teachers co-ordinating the 'special' work in schools. So too, the close co-operation of parents, teachers and other professionals in working together towards success for the child. In the end, however, the crucial factors are likely to be in the hands of the individual teacher as she prepares to face her class (further discussions on the Warnock Report are given in Booth and Potts, 1983; and Barton and Tomlinson, 1981).

The 1981 Act: Basic Duties of the LEA

The new education law which came into force on 1 April 1983, its Regulations, and the government circulars which consider the implications of the Act, all advise education authorities about the new procedures in special education. Many of the ideas and arguments put forward by the Warnock Committee have been put into effect. Schools have a duty to be more generally aware of the importance of recognising special needs. The details of the legislation cover the more specific duties and powers regarding identification and assessment, particularly the involvement of parents in the process. There are major changes in the way in which parental views and rights are taken into account by the LEA. But the responsibilities of parents are also recognised in ensuring that their child takes part in the processes of assessment, if the LEA insists, and in co-operating with any agreed plan of treatment. Wherever practicable, children are to be educated 'in accordance with the wishes of their parents'. School governors are given the duty of ensuring that the special needs already identified for a particular child are made known to those who teach the child, *and* provided for; whilst the LEA must keep any special arrangements under review. The most basic duty which has been placed upon the LEA is to ensure that adequate educational opportunities are available to all children, including those with special needs.

The 1981 Act: Which Children?

Under the new legislation a child has special educational needs if he or she has a learning difficulty which calls for special educational provision to be made. A child has a learning difficulty if he or she has 'significantly greater difficulty in learning than the majority of children of his age'. This is also described in the Act as 'a disability which either prevents or hinders him from making use of educational facilities of a kind generally provided in schools, within the area of the local authority concerned, for children of his age. Children under 5 can be considered if they are *likely* to have difficulties later on. However, a child is not to be taken as having a learning difficulty simply because the language used at home is different from that used in school.

The concept of special need under the new Act is a very broad one, following on Warnock, and a large number of children come within its terms of reference. Every school is likely to have some children with special needs. However, not all of this group will require *formal* assessment by the LEA to decide on provision to be made. Most LEAs will have existing arrangements for identifying children in need of special help, and a range of specialist services and facilities which the ordinary school can call on for advice. Almost all schools can call on a nurse, doctor, educational psychologist, specialist teachers of reading or of the hearing-impaired, perhaps a speech therapist or physiotherapist, for support. Local resources will vary greatly, but this wider group of children with special needs may well be helped within the normal arrangements made by the LEA to support the ordinary schools: a part of the 'continuum of provision' suggested by Warnock.

All hearing-impaired children, *ipso facto*, have special needs. At the very least, a child with a minor hearing-loss is *hindered* in his learning, and his progress should be monitored. This might take the form of a visiting specialist teacher calling into the ordinary school once a term to check on the child's progress. Under the Act this is an informal arrangement usually possible within the resources already available to the schools. The child has special needs in the broadest sense of Warnock, but is unlikely to require the full involvement of the multi-professional team.

A Right to Integration?

We have already suggested that integration can never be an end in itself, since the aims of education, the teaching objectives, remain the same, however these are achieved. Integration is a process, not a goal. The thinking behind the new legislation also tries to get rid of some other false assumptions. It is sometimes thought that children who are integrated into ordinary schools are those who would otherwise be in special schools or units. If we accept the wider concept of special need, integration is not an either/or question, but simply the process of helping children with varying degrees of special need within the context of an ordinary school.

The 1981 Act places a general duty on LEAs to help as many children as possible who have special needs within the ordinary school. Children cannot be excluded because of the nature of their handicap, whether physical, sensory or intellectual, or because of its severity, and provided the parents' views have been taken into account. Having said that, there are several major conditions which must be satisfied. The Act is not a charter for closing all special schools and admitting every child into mainstream education. Nevertheless, the spirit of the law is towards supporting integration wherever possible.

What are the conditions under which integration should take place? The Act says that education within the ordinary school must be compatible with the child receiving the special help he requires. Furthermore, this should not interfere with providing 'efficient education' for the *ordinary* majority of children. Where integration takes place this should represent an 'efficient use of resources'. Finally, there are some general guidelines to those responsible for special needs to make sure that such children are able 'to associate in the activities of the school with other children'.

For the hearing-impaired child the practice of placing children in units with access to mainstream schools is already well established, especially with younger age groups. It seems unlikely that the new legislation, *per se*, will commit local authorities to developing *new* schemes for integrating special-needs children or for changes in existing policy.

There is then, much room for interpretation. Parents have been given the right to *ask* for their child to be considered in terms of integration with ordinary children. We have argued that for hearing-impaired children there can be no rigid, all-encompassing solutions. A whole range of factors has to be weighed one against the other for every child. And for those children who are considered for some form of mainstream classroom help, the day to day 'ups and downs' have then to be negotiated. Furthermore, we have a responsibility to ensure that whatever arrangements are made under the 'umbrella' of integration, the child's experience socially, emotionally and academically, is carefully evaluated over time.

Informal Procedures

The most complex proposals in the Act concern procedures whereby a formal assessment of a child's special needs is made, leading to a 'statement'. However, the accompanying Circular 1/83 offers much advice to LEAs about children at the stages *before* formal assessments are made. Again there are wider duties to collect and record information about children, to begin consultation with parents as early as possible and to seek relevant professional help.

The Circular suggests, in reflecting another Warnock principle, that schools should shift their focus away from children's disabilities to the children themselves. A child's special needs are as much related to his strengths as his weaknesses, to the personal qualities and resources of the child, as well as to the support he gets at home and in school. Assessment of these interrelated factors is an ongoing process aimed at a better understanding of the child and how he can be helped. This process will usually begin, for the child of school age, with the ordinary classteacher. In the government Circular which accompanies the Act, LEAs have been advised to issue guidance to all schools on the local arrangements for 'identifying, assessing and meeting special educational needs'. Teachers and parents can therefore ask to see copies of any information relating to referral procedures, whom to turn to for advice, which specialist services are available, and so on. Normally, if a classteacher is concerned about a child, or a parent expresses worries, the headteacher of the school should be the first to be told. Where, for example, a teacher *becomes* concerned at a child's hearing, the headteacher should be consulted, who will then decide what steps to take next.

The Circular describes what it calls 'a progressive extension of professional involvement' starting with the classteacher, then the head, a visiting specialist teacher such as a remedial reading expert, on to the educational psychologist, school doctor and so on. The lines of communication between the school and outside agencies must be clear and effective. At this stage if a child is recognised as having special needs the educational implications must be known by the teacher and the parent. There must be close co-operation between the different parties, and easy access to appropriate help and advice before situations become critical. The Circular also advises that teachers should keep full records of their pupils' progress and notes about any professional consultations and assessments. It suggests that schools should be frank and open with parents, but there is to date no statutory obligation on teachers to allow parents to see their own children's records. Most LEAs have already evolved their own systems of screening and record keeping for children in school, which are a part of the informal procedures under the Act.

The Teacher's Own Assessment

What kind of observations can the teacher make upon a hearing-impaired child in the ordinary class? Unequivocally, those who spend long periods with a child, in different situations and over time, can come to a very clear view of the child's functioning, achievements in basic-skill areas, social relationships, interaction with others, general confidence, maturity, and so forth.

Teachers sometimes get very anxious when the performance of hearing-impaired children in their classes does not match up to their hearing peers. In comparison with ordinary children, the achievements of some hearing-impaired youngsters may seem very poor. There are two points of reassurance that should be made. First, the achievements of the hearing-impaired child in the ordinary school may be considerably better than could be reached in an alternative placement, such as a special school. Secondly, and more importantly, given the obstacles to learning and development which even a moderate hearing-loss presents, we should think in terms of how well the child is progressing in face of his difficulties.

In order to help structure teachers' observations we have devised several assessment frameworks for non-specialist teachers to use. These were prepared so that consistent samples of a child's progress in particular skill areas could be taken, which can then form the basis of an ongoing assessment record over a long period of time. The schedules are also helpful in planning appropriate teaching and learning objectives for a specific child. We have, throughout this book, stressed the appropriateness of careful prior planning of what the teacher sets out to do in her class teaching, and what she hopes the child will achieve. This is important, not only so that the hearing-impaired child can be prepared for the class experience and subsequently reinforced by support staff, but also to form an objective basis against which the child's learning can be evaluated.

At various age levels we have outlined the way in which specific objectives can be written and what areas of learning, in terms of skills or subject content, the child should have mastered at the end of the teaching process. Where objectives are thought out carefully, the processes of planning, monitoring and re-evaluating the child's educational programme are intrinsically linked. In terms of the 1981 Education Act, the ongoing monitoring which we hope teachers will carry out, is part of the informal assessment process. It may arise out of the assessment 'partnership' between teachers, parents and professionals, that a child is felt to have a complex or severe learning difficulty. It is at this point that it may be appropriate to give the child the 'protection' of a statement by initiating the *formal* procedures under the Act. Indeed, many hearing-impaired children will already be 'statemented' having gone through formal procedures earlier on. The details regarding formal reporting on children with special needs are dealt with separately. They will in fact depend very much on the kind of information that the classteacher has collected over time, using measures such as the ones we put forward.

Profiles of the Hearing-impaired (PHI)

The PHI charts aim to give detailed descriptions of a particular child's skills and abilities in the most relevant areas of development, according to the demands of the pre-school or school context. So for the very young child the focus is almost exclusively on communication, whereas emphasis broadens in later stages to include a wider sampling of academic attainment and social skills. These are not tests in the sense that items can be passed or failed, neither are they exhaustive; simply a means of shaping the teacher's observations as a prelude to setting realistic teaching objectives.

Figure 6.1: Profile of the Hearing-impaired (PHI) — Early Language Skills

Name
Date of Birth
Date of Assessment

Non-verbal Communication   (Tick as appropriate)
Looks at face of person speaking
Smiles as an appropriate response
Localises source of sound (telephone, doorbell)
Sustains eye-contact with speaker
Reaches out to be lifted up
Shakes head for 'No'
Shows recognition of everyday object (shoe, brush, cat)
Points at objects
Pulls person to get attention to show toys
Uses simple gestures to make needs known (toilet, drink)

Focuses attention on an activity for a few seconds
Uses a complex range of gestures including facial expressions
Needs adult help to sustain attention for 30 seconds or more
Able to concentrate on a task without help
Appropriate play with large toys (pots and pans, pram)
Uses small toys in play (cars, animals)
Enjoys pretend play (tea-set, dressing up, telephones, doctors and nurses)
Looks at a picture book

Understanding of Language
Quietens to noise
Recognises familiar voices (mother, grandma)
Understands commands such as 'No', 'Hot'
Responds to own name
Shows situational understanding (time for bed, clap hands, give Daddy a kiss, do your nappie)
Can indicate a named object (ball, teddy, book)
Follows simple commands (give to daddy, get your cup)
Points to parts of his body (hair, eyes, tummy)
Follows two-part directions (give the shoe to baby)
Can select objects by use (which do we drink with?)
Identifies object-function in pictures (show me the one that flies, which can we eat?)
Responds appropriately to simple sentences including:
1. Location words (in, on, under)
2. 'Doing' words (run, jump, sleep, cry)
3. Describing words (big, fat, hard, dirty)
4. Possessives (mine, daddy's, baby's, the dog's)
5. Time (now, tomorrow, later)
Responds appropriately to complex sentences including:
1. Questions (whose?, where?, why?)
2. Negatives (not, won't, isn't)
3. Comparatives (bigger, happiest, quietest)

Spoken Language
Vocalises (laughing, gurgling)
Babble combinations (baba, dada)
Babble strings (ga da ma)
Imitates sounds of objects (moo cow, brm brm)
Talks in jargon with intonation
Has a few words (dada, dolly, gee gee)
Has a spoken vocabulary of 20-30 words
Uses 50 clear words
Puts 2 words together (daddy gone)
Uses pronouns (I, me)
Uses 5-10 verbs
Puts 3 words together (mummy gone work)
Talks in simple sentences
Accompanies play with talking aloud

Uses language to plan and direct play
Uses language to interact with others
Uses more complex sentences and connecting devices such as 'and', 'because', 'but'

Give an example of a typical utterance:
What has been found to be particularly helpful in stimulating interaction and communication?
Give brief details of the child's aids and their use:

Figure 6.2: Profile of the Hearing-impaired (PHI) — the Junior Child

Name
Date of Birth
Date of Assessment

Hearing and Speech   (Tick as appropriate)
Shows reluctance at wearing hearing-aid
Able to replace aid in ear and take care of batteries
When using radio aids alerts teacher to any problems
Listens well in quiet 1- to-1 situations only
Comprehension of vocabulary is restricted and shows many gaps and confusions
Language interaction is limited to adult/child situations
Child's expressive speech is mostly labelling
Poor articulation means that child is difficult to understand out of context
Listens to a story in a small group for 10 minutes or so
Can demonstrate comprehension of simple instructions
Enjoys conversation with another child or adult
Has control of simple sentence patterns in speech
Child's speech can be understood by strangers out of context although articulation is affected
Listens to and demonstrates comprehension of oral instructions in large teaching groups
Has a wide vocabulary of everyday objects and activities
Can enter the 'to and fro' of conversation in group situations
Child's expressive speech is clearly articulated and shows complex sentence structures
Child understands language in the abstract and to refer out of context or beyond the 'here and now'

Give an example of a typical utterance:
Any specific problem situations which have arisen, or particularly helpful strategies for communication?
What does the teacher need to do differently?

Social Skills
Plays alongside rather than with other children
Shows anxiety at new situations or unfamiliar people
Dependent on adults for basic needs such as securing toys, toilet, dressing, initiating activities
Has few playmates and is isolated in mainstream groups
In groups may be passive, reluctant or sensitive, particularly if asked to speak
Rarely approaches other children or asks for help spontaneously
Shows some frustrations or tantrums when thwarted
In the playground is included by hearing children in games
Shows some confidence and independence in basic self-help, such as asking for things at lunch-table
Generally positive and enthusiastic when asked to complete a task
Regularly has social contacts with hearing peers, such as in after-school clubs or at home
Relies on other children and imitates their behaviour, such as laughing when they do but not understanding the joke
Other children help out with communication needs or lesson supports in class
Shows confidence and enthusiasm alongside peers in PE, sport, and in the playground
Socially independent and well-adjusted for age

Specify respective amounts of integration/support child enjoys:
Where are social difficulties likely to arise?

Educational Achievements
Attention control is intermittent, sustained for a few seconds only
Needs small, well-defined tasks, frequent activity changes, reinforcement and checking
Teacher prompts are useful in formal tasks
Can work independently and with concentration levels expected of peer group

Enjoys picture books in reading
Has a sight vocabulary of a few familiar words
Can read aloud more than 20 words and build into sentences
Tackles new or unfamiliar words
Uses context clues to read sentences for meaning
Can take in a paragraph and answer comprehension questions
Monitors own errors in reading and self-corrects
Enjoys simple readers and can relate the story sequence
Reads for information using reference books, graphs, tables, maps, newspapers
Independently reads with understanding books appropriate to peer group

Has hand control required for cutting, drawing, threading, writing
In writing needs to copy letter by letter/word by word/a model sentence
Can spell 10 simple regular words from dictation
Attempts common irregular words

To write a sentence needs to be given a stem to complete, 'cloze' task, most of the words
Generates own sentences but needs to correct
Writes a short sequence of ideas and can locate words in dictionary
Creates own stories

Can count, read and write numbers up to 10
Basic addition and subtraction up to 20
Competent in the four arithmetic processes up to 30
Handles money and correct change
Uses concepts of size, weight, time, length, height
Measures and records using ruler, scales, clock
Can divide a set into fractions; add, subtract and divide fractions
Uses concepts such as more, same, longest, equal, below, highest, shorter

---

Specify child's reading book/level of reading:
Specify maths attainment in relation to peers:
Any particular problem areas of learning?
What kind of additional supports are needed?

Figure 6.3: Profile of the Hearing-impaired (PHI) — the Senior Child

Name
Date of Birth
Date of Assessment

Hearing and Speech   (Tick as appropriate)
Wears hearing-aid without embarrassment
Takes responsibility for hearing-aids (batteries, PE, swimming)
Sits in good listening positions in class without reminder
If using a radio aid checks proper functioning with teacher
Alerts teacher to difficult listening conditions, such as noise interference
Responds to key words and finds sentences difficult
Frequent need to check for gaps in understanding
Has control of simple grammatical sentences in speech
Difficulties in following instructions given orally
Where misunderstandings arise will attempt other strategies (such as re-phrasing, gesture, writing)
Points out to others that he/she doesn't understand
Needs help to phrase an answer to a question
Hearing children communicate effectively with child
Understands and uses a wide range of complex sentence structures
Talks freely about his or her deafness
Able to sustain attention for most of a lesson
Needs help to cope with subject changes (lesson plans, teaching content, technical vocabulary)

Listens selectively and can summarise main points or take notes

_____

Communication problems may arise in certain situations such as group discussions (specify):

Specify any particular strategies which work well with child, such as enabling lip-reading:

What does the teacher need to do differently?

Social Interaction

Is socially isolated in mainstream classes

Is embarrassed to speak in front of a group of hearing children

Mainly to be seen in the company of other hearing-impaired children

Other people avoid talking to the child because of communication problems

Makes friends with hearing peers

Has some coping strategies which betray poor understanding (puts hand up but doesn't know the answer)

Shows frustration when misunderstandings arise

Joins in extra-curricular activities in mainstream, such as chess club, gymnastics, art group

Easily upset by difficulties or changes in routine

Not afraid of informal gatherings with hearing children, such as playground, disco, snack bar

Aware of socially acceptable behaviour according to the situation — doesn't just follow others' leads

Keeps up with social trends in dress, hair-styles, music

Sees other people's points of view, not just his/her own

Confident and independent in organising day-to-day needs such as bus pass, time-table, books and materials, homework

Mature in sexual knowledge and attitudes

Addresses others appropriately, enters conversation at proper point, holds a sustained dialogue

Other hearing children find him/her an interesting and attractive companion

_____

Specify respective amounts of integration/support child enjoys:

Where are social difficulties likely to arise?

Study Skills

Is a word-by-word reader; tends to extract familiar words and guess the rest

Needs help to read simple sentences and vocabulary

Is a sentence reader — shows comprehension in completion or 'cloze'-type tasks

Can read a passage to locate a point of information or main idea

In written work needs to be given the sentence frame and vocabulary

Able to use contents, index, headings and summaries to gain information

Needs help with handwriting, laying-out and presentation of work

Spelling difficulties with common words (specify)

Can digest a paragraph of text and answer questions or make notes on content
The 'carrier' language of most textbooks is likely to be overwhelming
Able to copy accurately from work card, blackboard or textbook
Needs help to answer technical vocabulary, interpret maps, tables, figures, diagrams, graphs
Can read a story or text and relate the sequence of ideas or events
Generates written language without help to express opinions and feelings
Can assume mastery of complex language in reading, writing and vocabulary, for all but more specialised subject areas
Follows detailed instructions and able to work independently
Seeks information in dictionary, library, encyclopaedia and takes notes

---

Specify the kind of supports which child requires to participate in mainstream classes, such as lesson plans, tutorial work, preparation and reinforcement:

Formal Statutory Procedures

Circular 1/83 says that

> formal procedures should be initiated where there are prima facie grounds to suggest that a child's needs are such as to require provision additional to, or otherwise different from, the facilities and resources generally available in ordinary schools in the area under normal arrangements.

This will obviously vary from area to area depending on the kind of help schools can normally call upon. In some authorities where teachers of the hearing-impaired normally visit *all* schools, the child with mild hearing difficulties will not require the provision of *extra* resources to that which is already available to ordinary schools in the area.

However, the child who requires a weekly visit from a peripatetic teacher, where this is not normally available, the child who may be supported in other ways such as additional classroom help to that already available, or the child who requires help for at least part of the time from a unit for the hearing-impaired, should all have the protection of a formal statement.

The key factor is that such help is not normally available to the ordinary school. As a general rule, *all* children in special units, special schools or approved independent schools, will be given statements. Where the help is provided from the ordinary school's own resources, where it involves a reading centre or disruptive unit, where the need for help is of short duration, or by agreement with the parent involves temporary placement in a special school as part of the assessment process, then formal statements are not required. Obviously, many of the hearing-impaired children we have discussed in this book will already have 'statements'.

The exact point at which a local education authority decides to start the formal statutory procedures will depend on the nature and severity of the child's needs, and the quality of existing resources within the area of the school. In any case, if the school has fulfilled its duty to consult with parents as early as possible, to seek professional advice where necessary, and to be frank and open about children's problems, then the initiation of formal procedures will not come as a surprise to any of the parties involved. In practice, there ought to have been much discussion, thought, often assessments carried out, before this point is reached.

Parents themselves can request a formal assessment for their child. Under the age of 2 years a local authority's duties to identify and provide for children apply *only with* parental consent. Formal arrangements including the making of statements, apply to children over the age of 2 years. If a parent requests a multi-professional assessment and the officers within the local authority feel the request is 'unreasonable', then the request can be turned down, leaving the parents the right of appeal against the decision. If a child is already subject to a statement but the last full assessment was 6 months ago, the parents can request another formal assessment. Again the authority can decide that this would be inappropriate, leaving the parent with the right of appeal.

Proposal to Assess

In some authorities it will usually only be after consultation between the parent, headteacher, educational psychologist, or medical officer, where appropriate, that a proposal for formal assessment is made. They will already have shared the concern over the child's progress or future difficulties. The LEA is required under the Act to notify the parents in writing that a full assessment is to be made. Usually, the parents should be given information about the procedures to be followed, what is entailed, and what the legal rights and duties are. Many authorities have produced booklets setting out the detailed arrangements, the kind of policies adopted locally, the nature of facilities and resources available, where to obtain further information, and so on.

Importantly, at this stage the parents are given the right to make representations about the proposal to assess within 29 days of being notified. If the parent objects to the proposal by writing to the LEA within this period, the reasons for any objection will be considered. Parents who want help in making their views known can ask for this through a 'named officer'. Parents may use their own initiatives at this early stage and gather support from say, the GP, Health Visitor, sympathetic teacher, independent psychologist, or whoever else will support a case for *not* assessing the child. After the 29-day period, the authority then decides whether to go ahead with a full assessment or not, and the parents are informed in writing. Parents can appeal to the Secretary of State about the proposal, but it is unlikely that the process can be halted if the local authority still wishes to assess.

Multi-professional Assessment

The 1981 Act lays down that at least four people must give their views about a child's special needs. Parents are asked what they feel about their child's difficulties and what kind of help they would prefer. In some authorities the child's headteacher supplies a form for the parents to complete, which is later appended to the formal statement of the child's needs. The authority must take into account any other evidence submitted by the parents, including any representations made at the proposal stage.

A second contributor to the full assessment process must be someone capable of giving educational advice. For pre-school children this may be a visiting teacher who knows the child, such as a specialist teacher counsellor for the mentally handicapped. In many cases this will be the headteacher of the child's school, who will obviously wish to consult with those teachers who have direct contact with the child in the classroom before the educational viewpoint is given. The kind of advice requested and how this can best be presented to help the child, is dealt with later in this chapter. For a few children, such as those felt to be significantly hearing or visually handicapped, advice should be sought from teachers qualified to teach the hearing or visually impaired.

A third contributor must be qualified to give medical advice about the child so that any medical problems likely to affect the child's educational needs are known. This will often be the school doctor. A fourth and final contribution to the full assessment, as a basic minimum requirement, must be given by an educational psychologist. In some situations, such as for the hearing-impaired, there may be a specialist educational psychologist who is asked to examine a child so that as full a picture as possible can be drawn up. So too, if the child has been seen in a hospital or assessment unit there may be several psychologists' views to take into account.

There may well be other people whose advice is called upon, such as a speech therapist, physiotherapist, psychiatrist or audiologist. In many cases the child is already known to these people, and any advice they give will be based on both past and present knowledge of the child. The Act also requires LEAs to ask both local nursing and social services if they know of any difficulties which the child may have. In some cases each professional adviser will send advice separately to the authority. There may well be case conferences when those involved will get together to share, discuss and harmonise their views. Parents can ask to attend such meetings, but have no legal right to do so.

The parents do have a right, however, to be informed of any examinations which are going to be made of their child by professionals such as doctors or psychologists. The notice must state the time, place and purpose of the examination, as well as outlining parental rights to be present and where to get further information from. If the child is not presented for examination and there is no reasonable excuse, the parents can be taken to court and fined up to £50.

What Kind of Advice?

The 1981 Act and the circulars which accompany it, set out fairly clearly the kind of advice required from the professionals contributing to the formal procedures. Since the ordinary classteacher with day-to-day familiarity with the child is in a key position to give an educational view of the child, much of what teachers have to say about a child's needs will, either directly or indirectly, appear on the final statement. It is highly important, therefore, that teachers are aware of their role in giving educational advice, and know the kind of information which is most helpful to give. In general, the role of the professional contributors is to analyse and set out the child's special needs, and suggest practical approaches to meet them. It is not part of the adviser's role to give the name of a suitable school placement. Nor should knowledge of local resources influence the nature of the advice given. At this stage the child's profile of special needs and the *specific* educational provision the authority will make to meet them, are quite separate issues from each other.

The new Act has adopted the ideas put forward by Warnock regarding the main focus of advice about a child. The practice of fitting children up with labels such as ESN(M) is unacceptable. We can only arrive at a better understanding of the child himself by building up a picture of individual strengths and weaknesses. We need relevant and known facts about the child's environment, his history, his home, his relationships with other children, his functioning in school. Value judgements are to be avoided. Emotive language can be misleading and misinterpreted. It must be remembered that under the terms of the new Act, the professional advice given to the LEA is copied verbatim in the appendices to the formal statement, is available to the parents to see, and in the event of an appeal, to the appeal committee.

Some consideration has already been given to the teacher's careful record-keeping over time, using a clear framework of observation. The PHI charts provide a model for detailing a profile of the child's abilities and deficiencies, in an informal way, and which provide a foundation for planning teaching objectives. It is precisely this kind of depiction of what the child has achieved educationally and what the future teaching programme should aim to achieve, which is required by the formal procedures.

The local authority may in fact provide teachers and headteachers with guidelines in preparing written reports on children. The Warnock idea is that assessment is an ongoing process whereby every school compiles information over time regarding children's development, which is discussed honestly with parents. So schools might be asked to look back in their records to comment on the time when problems first became apparent, which agencies were contacted and when, what arrangements were made for the child before the assessment procedure was formalised and whether these were successful, when significant home factors arose, whether school attendance has been good, and what factors have led up to the present need for a statutory statement of needs.

There will certainly be amongst any such guidelines to teachers, a very large emphasis upon the child's level of skill in areas relevant to education. Literacy, numeracy and general communication skills are, of course, highly important. It is here that teachers need to be as specific as possible, sticking closely to what they have observed and measured in the child, rather than intuited. The details of any tests should be given with the date of administration.

For the child in school with a handicap such as cerebral palsy, visual deficit or hearing-impairment, certain aspects of the curriculum and of the physical environment of the school itself will pose greater problems than others. A child with cerebral palsy will be at greater risk in a laboratory or workshop than in a classroom. A visually handicapped child will have greater special needs in negotiating stairs but be comfortable in the swimming pool. A hearing-impaired child dependent on hearing-aids may find the assembly hall and football pitch overwhelmingly difficult situations to cope with, compared with the library or music room. Special needs arise uniquely for children depending on their handicaps, personal qualities and the situations they find themselves in. This kind of detailed description is absolutely necessary for our full understanding.

The headteacher in compiling a profile of the child's strengths and weaknesses will usually also be asked by the LEA to suggest ways in which practical help can be given to the child, the kind of curriculum which would be appropriate, and which aspects of the child's functioning need special attention. There may be physical needs which require independence training, specific intellectual skills or weaknesses, inadequate social skills, or a need to concentrate on aspects such as expressive language. The better the definition which is given to these special needs the more likely that provision can be made which is appropriate to meet them.

There is scope at this stage for teachers to suggest specific equipment, such as a radio aid, low-vision aid, rollator; to highlight special teaching methods which have been or could be useful, such as a language-based reading scheme, computer-aided teaching, behaviour-modification techniques; and to include other teaching resources which should be involved, such as help from a teacher of the hearing-impaired, speech therapist, or occupational therapist. It is most important to reiterate, at this stage, that the local authority should not be committed to any specific course of action such as a particular school or unit placement, since decision-making is a separate process.

The Statement

Following the assessment the LEA may or may not decide to make the child subject to a statement of special educational needs. If it does, regulations must be followed which detail the form and content. The statement should specify the Authority's view of the special educational needs of the child, having taken into account the views and advice of all concerned, including the parents. Copies of all the assessment documents submitted by advisers must be appended to the statement. The statement must also specify the special educational provision to be made for the child, the kind of resources, facilities and arrangements to be made to meet the child's needs. The kind of school considered to be appropriate for the child must be described and named, if known. Similarly, any other additional provisions to be made by health or social services should be set out.

There are two steps in the preparation of the statement. First, a proposed statement is drafted, usually in consultation with the professionals who submitted advice to the LEA. The Act requires the LEA to send a copy of the draft statement to the parents. Parents then have the right to make representations and to discuss the draft statement with an officer of the LEA. If the parents disagree with any part of the assessment they must inform the LEA within 15 days of the date the statement was issued. Further interviews may be arranged with professionals who contributed advice, such as the doctor or psychologist, if necessary. The parent should be given the opportunity to visit any named school under consideration.

At the second stage, after considering any parental views, the LEA then decides whether to make a statement in the form originally proposed, to make a modified statement or none at all. When a final statement is made a copy must be sent to the parents together with the notice of the right to appeal, and the name of an officer from whom further advice can be obtained. The date by which the child's progress and placement will be reviewed should also be given.

If the parent still disagrees with the LEA about a child's statement there are guidelines laid down for parental appeals. These are heard by special local committees, but in intractable situations the parent has the right of appeal to the Secretary of State for Education and Science who will make the final decision.

Reviews

The new Act requires LEAs to review statements at least once a year. Reviews will be prepared by the headteacher of the child's school based on reports from the classteacher and other professionals involved. The concept of ongoing assessment taken from Warnock underlies this process of frequent review and discussion between teachers, other professionals and parents. The first review of the child's progress and placement must take place within 12 months of the date on which the final statement is issued.

A full multi-professional reassessment of a child's needs may be made as a result of an annual review. This will involve, as a minimum, the four separate contributions outlined earlier. A parent can request a full reassessment after 6 months of the date of a final statement, but the Authority may decline this request. Full reassessments are normally only indicated where there has been 'a significant change in the circumstances of the child'. A local authority is obliged to reassess a child at one particular point: unless the original statement was made after the child was 12½ years, there must be a full reassessment between the ages of 13½ and 14½ years. The logic of this is to enable future planning for the child in his last years at school, to consider any vocational training, further education, or employment prospects. If, following reassessment, the LEA decides to change or discontinue a statement, parents must be informed in writing and have 15 days to make representations, with the right of appeal.

Some Implications

Different local education authorities will respond to the challenges of the new legislation in different ways. The full implications will be worked out over time, and through the courts, whose job it is, in the end, to make legal interpretations of the provisions of the Act. The immediate implications are obvious: a much greater involvement of parents in the process of consultation and assessment. Unfortunately, this is at the expense of a lengthy and complex bureaucratic process. For those parents who want their child to have special educational help and would prefer to leave the arrangements to others, the official aspects of the process may seem overwhelming and threatening. It is certainly time consuming given the statutory periods of notice, and the number of occasions on which written communications must pass between different agencies.

The intentions of the new law are laudable. The concept of 'special needs' replaces what many feel are offensive and stigmatising labels. The shift of focus away from the child's disability to a more objective view of both strengths and weaknesses, and the individuality of the child in his particular environment, is welcomed. If teachers are to work effectively with handicapped children in integrated classes teaching objectives must be made clear. We have argued in this book that clear target setting for children is the key to a co-ordinated programme when children are 'supported' in mainstream classes part-time. It is the basis for realistic evaluation of progress, and underlies the notion of ongoing review.

Integration, we have said, is not an end in itself, and this is supported in the new legislation. The Act asks LEAs to consider the integration of handicapped children in ordinary schools where this is practicable. Perhaps most importantly of all, the wider concept of special needs gets rid of the notion of integration being an either/or issue. Integration in ordinary schools is not an *alternative* to special-school placement. We have also argued in this book that for hearing-impaired children, as for any other disability, there needs to be as wide and flexible a range of educational opportunities available as possible: a continuum of provision, in Warnock terms, to meet every individual child's needs. Many of these needs of course, can be met by an educational programme which includes some contact with ordinary children.

The new Act by itself will not change the attitudes of society at large to the handicapped minority since that is not an issue which can be legislated for. However, the way to increase understanding must be through schools, where children with and without disabilities can live and work together positively. This is where the seeds of trust and acceptance are sown.

The new legislation makes no mention of any additional financial resources to LEAs in order to implement the principles of the Act. Many of the professionals contributing to the new procedures, particularly teachers, are going to find themselves with greater responsibilities to bear. We have also argued in this book that it is a mistake to ask the ordinary classteacher to share in making provision for children with difficulties, without ensuring that proper resources, training and advice are available. For hearing-impaired children we must not talk in terms of a reduction in the special help available, but of how and where this is given. In the end, of course, it is the ordinary classteacher who has the day-to-day challenge of providing a meaningful experience for a handicapped child within the classroom. Under the new Act LEAs have a responsibility to ensure that there are effective lines of communication, that schools have access to advice and close liaison with relevant professionals, and that once identified the child's special needs are met as far as possible. The annual review provides the classteacher with a safeguard in that if arrangements are not working well for the special child, the teacher, or the majority of children, there is a point at which any concerns can be expressed about the adequacy of provision.

There is a world of difference between an educational experience which is adequate and one which is successful. The thinking behind this book is towards the latter: careful discussion, thought, awareness and co-ordination of effort whenever a hearing-impaired child spends some of his time in mainstream classes.

To the Future

We can look forward to an increasing understanding of deafness, its aetiology, treatment and implications. Preventive medicine, such as therapeutic abortion and rubella immunisation of teenage girls, has already shown a reduction in the number of multiply-handicapped deaf babies. Hopefully, we can look forwards to the earlier diagnosis of hearing-losses when they occur. Audiology is a young science with exciting developments in computer-aided testing and screening techniques, particularly for very young children. So too, in medical intervention there is a growing awareness of the problems associated with minor hearing-losses, and ongoing research into possibilities such as artificial nerve implants which detect sound. Hearing-aid technology has begun to provide powerful, flexible and sophisticated amplification; whilst radio aids are becoming smaller, more refined and reliable.

But the most important developments for the hearing-impaired are less tangible: changes in outlook and opportunity for children and families, supported for the first time by the law. Many of the new principles and ideals have already flourished in the hands of dedicated and gifted classteachers. We hope this book has given encouragement to those who are not so sure!

APPENDIX I

Warning Signs and Symptoms of a Hearing-loss

1. Child often appears 'catarrhal', 'blocked-up', or is a mouth-breather and has frequent absences with coughs or colds.
2. Verbal reports or medical records give a history of ear infections or failed screening tests, particularly in winter months.
3. Child complains of ear-ache, 'popping ears' or fullness in the ear, or has a visible discharge from the ear.
4. Appears to daydream and drift off, or is more alert when positioned close to the teacher.
5. Watches the speaker's face for clues and has difficulty listening to a message given without situational or speaker clues, such as over a tape recorder.
6. Child may need to search visually for the source of a sound and is unable to locate sounds quickly.
7. Child's speech may be limited in structure or vocabulary, with omission of some sounds and confusions in others.
8. May need to sit nearer the TV than normal, or ask for the volume on the record player or tape deck to be turned up.
9. Is slow in reacting to verbal instructions, asks for repetition or watches other children's lead.
10. Misunderstands or gives inappropriate responses, particularly if a sequence of spoken instructions is given.
11. Speech may seem softer or fuzzier than usual.
12. Appears inattentive and restless, or distracts others, particularly when asked to listen for a protracted period.
13. Child may not turn immediately when called by name unless the teacher gives some visible signals.
14. Some irritability, atypical aggression, bad-tempered behaviour or more frequent upsets in school.
15. Little interest in following a story, especially in noisy conditions.
16. Pace of learning falls away periodically and attention span shortens, or child tires more quickly than normal.
17. Asks for much more individual help and explanation than usual, but may withdraw from social contact with other children.

18. Academic difficulties in verbal skills such as reading, particularly in establishing sound-symbol associations, sound blends, or in discriminating between sounds.

APPENDIX II

Some Facts and Fallacies about Deafness

TRUE   FALSE

1. Most profoundly hearing-impaired people have *some* hearing.
2. Children with severe deafness cannot learn to talk.
3. Hearing-aids cannot restore a person's hearing.
4. Hearing-impaired children can learn to lip-read as well as the normally hearing.
5. You cannot learn to drive a car if you are severely hearing-impaired.
6. Deafness prevents people from enjoying music.
7. Conductive deafness cannot be treated.
8. Monaural deafness does not make any difference to a child.
9. Hearing can fluctuate from one day to the next.
10. Sensori-neural deafness cannot be treated.
11. Children can have both conductive and nerve deafness at the same time.
12. The level of a child's hearing-loss can change from one sound pitch to another.
13. Hearing-aids can be adjusted to fit the shape of a child's audiogram.
14. Rubella during pregnancy no longer damages babies' hearing.
15. Hearing-impairment can be inherited.
16. A congenital hearing-loss is detectable at birth.
17. It is more likely that a child will learn to speak if deafness is acquired in infancy.
18. A percentage hearing-loss tells you how much hearing a person has.

TRUE   FALSE

19.   A child's audiogram tells you whether he will
      be able to learn to speak.
20.   Hearing-impaired children under-achieve in
      school.

ANSWERS

 1.   TRUE   There are very few hearing-impaired people who have no
              hearing at all. The majority will therefore benefit from
              making use of residual hearing and from hearing-aids.
 2.   FALSE   When deafness is diagnosed early (7 or 8 months), with
              good hearing-aids, expert teaching and advice, most
              children with severe hearing-losses can learn some
              useful speech.
 3.   TRUE   Hearing-aids can only amplify sound into the ears — they
              cannot make damaged ears better.
 4.   FALSE   Because normally hearing people usually have excellent
              understanding of language it is easier to lip-read what is
              being said.
 5.   FALSE   Hearing-impaired people develop good visual awareness,
              and often have lower car insurance premiums than
              normally hearing drivers.
 6.   FALSE   Many hearing-impaired people enjoy music and can
              detect rhythms. Some learn to play instruments.
 7.   FALSE   Conductive hearing difficulties can often be treated by
              medicine or surgery. However, the problem quite often
              returns and further treatment is required.
 8.   FALSE   Listening in noisy surroundings and locating the direc-
              tion of the sound can cause difficulties.
 9.   TRUE   It is a well-recognised feature of *Otitis media* that hear-
              ing can fluctuate from one day to the next.
10.   TRUE   There is no medical or surgical procedure which can help
              if a person has nerve deafness.
11.   TRUE   Where a child has a 'mixed' loss it should be possible to
              improve the hearing by clearing up the conductive com-
              ponent, but the sensori-neural loss will remain.
12.   TRUE   The level of hearing-loss is a measure of the child's
              ability to hear quiet or loud sounds compared with our
              own. It can change markedly from high-pitch to low-
              pitch sounds.

13. TRUE   To some extent. Modern hearing-aids can cut out certain
            frequencies and amplify others. If a child has good
            hearing for high but not for low-pitch sounds, hearing-
            aids without a cut-out would amplify all the sounds the
            same amount, and this would be very painful to the
            child in the high-frequency range.
14. FALSE   Fewer mothers catch rubella because of immunisation.
            But for those who do the disease can still cause deafness,
            blindness and heart defects.
15. TRUE   For many children there is no known cause of hearing-
            loss, but it *is* known that children in families where
            hearing-loss has occurred before, such as in grandparents,
            are at greater risk. Genetic counselling may reveal the
            possibilities of having a hearing-impaired child.
16. FALSE   Hearing-impairment is difficult to detect in babies
            although techniques such as the 'auditory response
            cradle' are being developed. Babies with deafness may
            seem normal and babble. Most parents feel something is
            wrong by about 7-8 months, and this is when distraction
            testing can be done.
17. TRUE   If a child has normal hearing, even for a short time, this
            experience is important for future progress. A hearing-
            loss acquired *after* the child had begun to learn to talk
            creates less severe and quite different problems.
18. FALSE   We have often heard people described as having a 40, 50
            or 60 percentage hearing loss. These are meaningless as
            measurements and should be disregarded.
19. FALSE   There is little relation between degree and quality of a
            child's hearing-loss and ability to learn to speak. This
            does not mean that an audiogram has no useful informa-
            tion to give.
20. TRUE   In some schools where there is little understanding of
    and   the nature of a hearing-impaired child's difficulties, and
    FALSE   poor teaching, then the child will not reach his poten-
            tial. Where schools have purpose, awareness and commit-
            ment, then many of the obstacles associated with deaf-
            ness can be surmounted.

REFERENCES

Ainscow, M. and Tweddle, D.M. (1979) *Preventing Classroom Failure: an Objectives Approach*, London, Wiley & Sons

Ballantyne, J. (1977) *Deafness*, 3rd edn, Edinburgh, Churchill Livingstone

Barton, L. and Tomlinson, S. (eds) (1981) *Special Education: Policy, Practices and Social Issues*, London, Harper & Row

Bax, M., Hart, H. and Jenkins, S. (1983) 'The Behaviour, Development and Health of the Young Child: Implications for Care', *British Medical Journal*, vol. 286, 4 June, 1793-6

Bench, J. and Bamford, J.M. (1979) *Speech Hearing Tests and the Spoken Language of Hearing-Impaired Children*, London, Academic Press

Bishop, J. and Gregory, S. (1983) 'Going to School', *Talk*, Winter issue

—— and —— (1984) 'Linking Home and School', *Talk*, Spring issue

Booth, T. (1983) 'Integrating Special Education', in T. Booth and P. Potts (eds), *Integrating Special Education*, Oxford, Blackwell, pp. 1-27

—— and Potts, P. (eds) (1983) *Integrating Special Education*, Oxford, Blackwell

Bradley, L. (1980) *Assessing Reading Difficulties: A Diagnostic and Remedial Approach*, London, Macmillan

—— and Bryant, P. (1978) 'Difficulties in Auditory Organisation as a Possible Cause of Reading Backwardness', *Nature*, *271*, 746-7

Brown, R. (1977) 'Introduction', in C.E. Snow and C.A. Ferguson (eds.), *Talking to Children*, Cambridge University Press, Cambridge

Carter, K. (1983) 'Breaking through the Barriers', *ILEA Contact*, 24 June

Catlin, F.I. (1978) 'Etiology and Pathology of Hearing Loss in Children', in F.N. Martin (ed.), *Pediatric Audiology*, Englewood Cliffs, Prentice-Hall, pp. 3-34

Chazan, M., Laing, A.F., Bailey, M.S. and Jones, G. (1980) *Some of our Children: The Early Education of Children with Special Needs*, London: Open Books

Cleave, S., Jowett, S. and Bate, M. (1982) . . . *And so to School: A Study of Continuity from Pre-school to Infant School*, Windsor, NFER-Nelson

Conrad, R. (1979) *The Deaf School Child*, London, Harper & Row

Cooper, J., Moodley, M. and Reynell, J. (1978) *Helping Language Development: A Developmental Programme for Children with Early Language Handicaps*, London, Edward Arnold

Cox, K. (1983) 'Sex, Adolescents and Schools', in G. Lindsay (ed.), *Problems of Adolescence in the Secondary School*, London, Croom Helm, pp. 126-60

Crystal, D. (1976) *Child Language, Learning and Linguistics*, London, Edward Arnold

—— Fletcher, P. and Garman, M. (1976) *The Grammatical Analysis of Language Disability*, London, Edward Arnold

Dalzell, J. and Owrid, H.L. (1976) 'Children with Conductive Deafness: A Follow-up Study', *British Journal of Audiology, 10*, 87-90

Davies, F.I. and Greene, T. (1982) 'Effective Reading: Using Pupil Resources for

Comprehension and Learning', *Remedial Education*, Vol. 17, no. 4

Davis, J. (1974) 'Performance of Young Hearing-impaired Children on a Test of Basic Concepts', *Journal of Speech and Hearing Research, 17*, 342-51

DES: Tabulation of returns on forms 21M and 7 (Schools) at Table 1 of Consultative Document SH(82)3: 'The Need for Rationalisation of Special School Provision for the Hearing-impaired', June 1982, and statistics from the same sources for 1982 and 1983

—— (1967) *Units for Partially Hearing Children*, Education Survey No. 1, HMSO

——(1975) *A Language for Life*, (The Bullock Report) HMSO

—— (1978) *Primary Education in England*, HMSO

Downs, M.P. (1977) 'The Expanding Imperatives of Early Identification', in F. Bess (ed.), *Childhood Deafness: Causation, Assessment and Management*, New York, Grune & Stratton

Ewing, I.R. and Ewing, A.W.G. (1944) 'The Ascertainment of Deafness in Infancy and Early Childhood; *Journal of Laryngology and Otology, 59*, 309

Fundudis, T., Kolvin, I. and Garside, R. (eds) (1979) *Speech Retarded and Deaf Children: Their Psychological Development*, London, Academic Press

Gregory, S. (1976) *The Deaf Child and his Family*, London, George Allen & Unwin

—— and Mogford, K. (1981) 'Early Language Development in Deaf Children', in B. Woll, J. Kyle, and M. Deuchar (eds), *Perspectives on British Sign Language and Deafness*, London, Croom Helm, pp. 218-37

Hamblin, D.H. (1981) *Teaching Study Skills*, Oxford, Basil Blackwell

Harris, J. (1984) 'Early Language Intervention Programmes: An Update', *Association for Child Psychology and Psychiatry Newsletter*, vol. 6, no. 2, 2-20

Hegarty, S. and Pocklington, K. (1981) *Educating Pupils with Special Needs in the Ordinary School*, Windsor, NFER-Nelson

—— and —— (1982) *Integration in Action*, Windsor, NFER-Nelson

Hogg, B. (1984) *Microcomputers and Special Educational Needs: A Guide to Good Practice*, Stratford-upon-Avon, National Council for Special Education

Jeffree, D. and McConkey, R. (1983) *Let me Speak*, Human Horizons Series, Tiptree, Essex, Souvenir Press

Jones, E. (1981) 'A Resource Approach to Meeting Special Needs in a Secondary School', in L. Barton and S. Tomlinson (eds), *Special Education: Policy, Practices and Social Issues*, London, Harper & Row, pp. 212-34

Lindsay, G. (ed.) (1983) *Problems of Adolescence in the Secondary School*, London, Croom Helm

Lunzer, E. and Gardner, K. (eds) (1979) *The Effective Use of Reading*, London, Heinemann, for Schools Council

Manning, K. and Sharp, A. (1977) *Structuring Play in the Early Years at School*, London, Ward Lock Educational

Martin, F.N. (ed.) (1978) *Pediatric Audiology*, New Jersey, Prentice-Hall

Meadow, K.P. (1980) *Deafness and Child Development*, London, Edward Arnold

Mindel, E.D. and Vernon, M. (1971) *They Grow in Silence*, Silver Spring, Maryland, National Association of the Deaf

Murphy, K.P. (1976) in H.H. Oyer (ed.), *Communication for the Hearing Handicapped* Baltimore, University Park Press, 171

National Deaf Children's Society (1980) *Public Examinations and Hearing-*

Impaired Students, Report and Conclusions of a Survey by the Education Sub-committee

Quigley, S.P. (1978) 'Effects of Early Hearing-impairment on Normal Language Development', in F.N. Martin (ed.), *Pediatric Audiology*, New Jersey, Prentice-Hall, pp. 35-63

—— , Power, D. and Steinkamp, M. (1977) 'The Language Structure of Deaf Children', *Volta Review, 79*, 73-84

—— and Kretschmer, R.E. (1982) *The Education of Deaf Children: Issues, Theory and Practice*, London, Edward Arnold

Ross, M. (1982) *Hard of Hearing Children in Regular Schools*, Englewood Cliffs, New Jersey, Prentice-Hall

Rutter, M., Graham, P., Chadwick, O.F.D. and Yule, W. (1976) 'Adolescent Turmoil: Fact or Fiction', *Journal of Child Psychology and Psychiatry*, vol. 17, no. 1, 35-56

—— Maughan, B., Mortimore, P. and Ouston, J. (1979) *Fifteen Thousand Hours*, London, Open Books

—— Tizard, J. and Whitmore, K. (1970) *Education, Health and Behaviour*, London, Longman

Shah, N. (1981) 'Surgical Treatment of Conductive Deafness in Children', in H.A. Beagley (ed.), *Audiology and Audiological Medicine*, vol. 2, Oxford, Oxford University Press, p. 699

Snow, C.E. and Ferguson, C.A. (eds) (1977) *Talking to Children: Language Input and Acquisition*, Cambridge, Cambridge University Press

Swann, W. (1983) 'Curriculum Principles for Integration', in T. Booth and P. Potts (eds), *Integrating Special Education*, Oxford, Blackwell, pp. 100-24

Tizard, B. (1975) *Early Childhood Education: A Review and Discussion of Current Research in Britain*, Slough, NFER

Tough, J. (1973) *Focus on Meaning: Talking to Some Purpose with Young Children*, London, Allen & Unwin

—— (1977) *The Development of Meaning: A Study of Childrens' use of Language*, London, George Allen & Unwin

Tumin, W. (1978) 'Parents' Views', *Education Today*, Summer

Warnock Report (1978) *Special Educational Needs*, HMSO

Webb, L. (1974) *Purpose and Practice in Nursery Education*, Oxford, Blackwell

Webster, A. (In press) *Survival Skills*, Banbury, Burrough Press

—— and Danks, V. (1978) *Footsteps 1*, Edinburgh, Holmes McDougall

—— Saunders, E. and Bamford, J.M. (1984) 'Fluctuating Conductive Hearing-impairment', *Journal of the Association of Educational Psychologists*, in press

—— Wood, D.J. and Griffiths, A.J. (1981) 'Reading Retardation or Linguistic Deficit? I: Interpreting Reading Test Performances of Hearing-impaired Adolescents', *Journal of Research in Reading, 4*, 2, 136-47

Wells, G. (1979) 'Describing Children's Linguistic Development at Home and at School', *British Educational Research Journal* vol. 5, 1, 75-99

Westmacott, E.M.V. and Cameron, R.J. (1981) *Behaviour can Change*, Basingstoke, Globe Education

White, M. and East, K. (1981) 'Selecting Objectives in Language', *Remedial Education*, vol. 16, no. 4, 171-8

Wood, D.J. (1982) 'Fostering Language Development in Hearing-impaired

Children', in M.M. Clark (ed.), *Special Educational Needs and Children Under Five*, Educational Review Occasional Publications No. 9, University of Birmingham, pp. 20-5

—— McMahon, L. and Cranstoun, Y. (1980) *Working with Under-fives*, London, Grant McIntyre Ltd

—— Wood, H.A. and Howarth, S.P. (1983) 'Mathematical Abilities in Deaf School Leavers', *British Journal of Developmental Psychology* (in press)

Wood, H.A. and Wood, D.J. (1984) 'An Experimental Evaluation of the Effects of Five Styles of Teacher Conversation on the Language of Hearing-impaired Children, *Journal of Child Psychology and Psychiatry, 25*, 45-62

INDEX

Wood, H.A. 75, 89
writing 87-8, 130-2

Yule, W. 120

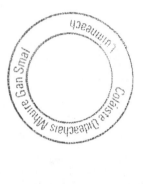